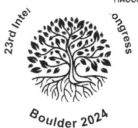

# Proceedings
## of the
# 23rd International Balint Congress

September 9-13, 2024
Boulder, Colorado, USA

## Cultivating Understanding and Compassion Through Balint

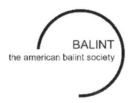

BALINT
the american balint society

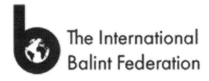

The International
Balint Federation

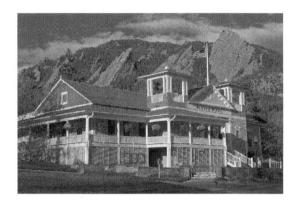

The Colorado Chautauqua
900 Baseline Road
Boulder, CO 80302  USA
www.chautauqua.com

Chief Editor, Karen Carlson
Published by the American Balint Society
August 2024
Copyright ©2024
All rights reserved
ISBN 9798329011180

## Congress Planning Committee

Allison Bickett, Co-Chair
E. Katherine Knowlton, Co-Chair
Shantel Beckers
Karen Carlson
Barbara Hemmendinger
Albert Lichtenstein
Donald Nease
Deborah Seymour
Brian Wexler

## Scientific Committee

Karen Carlson, Chair
Vidush Athyal
Eddo De Lang
Guido Flatten
E. Katherine Knowlton
Jessica Leão
Eran Metzger
Laurel Milberg
Lisa Whitten

# CONTENTS

# Introduction to the Proceedings

The American Balint Society is pleased to publish the Proceedings of the 23rd International Balint Congress taking place in Boulder, Colorado in September 2024. This book contains all the papers presented at the Congress, a selection of some of the papers submitted but not presented, and the abstracts of posters presented. It includes an overview of the workshops taking place in Boulder. While these depend heavily on experiential learning and are thus hard to convey, we wish to communicate their breadth and originality. You will also find the full text of papers selected for the 2024 ASCONA Prize awarded to students, whose fresh eyes and devotion to patient relationships remind us of why we may be drawn to Balint work or even to medicine itself. Taken as a whole, these Proceedings reflect some of the recent scholarship and creative efforts of members of the Balint community worldwide.

Woven through the body of work presented here is the theme of this year's Congress: Cultivating Understanding and Compassion Through Balint. Whether topics focused on unexpected strengths of Balint work, such as support for ethics or applicability to nonhuman medicine, or possible limits, such as discontinuing in a time of war, the authors showed understanding beyond the ordinary. We are confident that thoughtful acquaintance with these papers will help people deepen their own understanding of the field.

We would like to thank the contributors for sharing their research about Balint group work, their reflections about doing groups in new settings, and their ideas about how Balint groups can transform our thinking about creating meaningful professional relationships. We are grateful to the Organizing Committee for creating the framework in which Balint enthusiasts from around the world could gather to exchange ideas and cross-pollinate their work. Special thanks are due to the Scientific Committee for the significant time and attention they gave to review papers, workshops, and posters. We also thank the American Balint Society and the International Balint Federation for their many months of unflagging support. Finally, executive administrator Shantel Beckers deserves profound acknowledgement for her inestimable contribution to this event at every stage.

Our hope is that those who attend the Congress and others with an interest in learning more about Balint group work worldwide will find rich food for thought and fresh inspiration in these Proceedings.

Karen Carlson, MD
Chair, Scientific Committee
Congress Planning Committee
American Balint Society

# Introduction to the Congress

On behalf of the American Balint Society, it is my great pleasure to extend a warm and heartfelt welcome to each of you. When I was granted the privilege of becoming president of the American Balint Society, one of the first things I realized was that the International Balint Congress would be held in the United States during my term. What a bonus! I eagerly awaited the day when I could welcome Balint enthusiasts from around the world. That day has arrived, and I couldn't be more thrilled to see such a diverse and dedicated group gathered here.

I am excited to witness the fruition of over a year of meticulous planning by the organizing committee. They have chosen a stunning venue, solicited outstanding papers and workshops, and developed a timely theme: "Cultivating Compassion and Understanding through Balint."
This gathering represents a unique opportunity for us to come together, share our experiences, and deepen our understanding of the invaluable work we do. Your presence here is a testament to your commitment to fostering compassion and enhancing relationships in the medical and therapeutic fields.

Imagine if world leaders sought to cultivate compassion. Imagine if their meetings were focused on seeking deeper understanding through empathy, setting aside political and other divisive positions. That's what we have the opportunity and expectation to do here. However, we also come with our own differences, divisions, and biases. We are challenged to set aside these differences and move beyond our preconceived ways of seeing things.

I believe the values that draw us to Balint and the spirit of its method provide the buoyancy necessary to overcome these challenges. I am confident we can create an atmosphere of safety and respect, one in which we can express diverse ideas without judgment or criticism. It is this atmosphere that will keep us aligned with the theme of this gathering.

I encourage you all to fully engage in the sessions, workshops, and conversations that will unfold. Share your cases, ask questions, and be open to the perspectives of others.

Once again, welcome to the International Balint Federation Congress. Let us embark on this journey of compassion and understanding with open hearts and minds, ready to learn, grow, and make a lasting impact.

Thank you, and here's to an inspiring and transformative meeting!

Phillip A. Phelps, LCSW, President of the American Balint Society merican Balint Society

# Introduction to the Congress

It is an honour for me as president of the IBF to welcome all of you to this 23rd International Balint Federation Congress in Boulder under the theme of 'Cultivating understanding and compassion through Balint.' I'm going to take you through part of a session in a Balint group to illustrate some thoughts about the role of the conductor, the influence of the relationship, and how to keep the group in mind.

And then some of my actual reflections on how to start a group, and the meaning of the frame as a tool to stabilise the group and help the group contain the differences and diversities that are present among the members.

In the end I shall try to illustrate how this influences the development of a Balint group leader, from being in to belonging in a group. I talk about the group conductor and/or group leader, the similarities and differences between the roles.

### The role of the conductor in the group

The title is "The role of the conductor in the group". It could perhaps as well have been "The role of the group in the conductor," by this indicating the close and interwoven relationship between the way the conductor is present in the group and how it "gestalts" itself in his mind.

Let me start with a citation you all know by heart, placed in the very beginning of Appendix 1 (in Michael Balint's book, *The Doctor, the Patient, and the Illness*) about training[1]:

> The only way to acquire a new skill is to expose oneself to the actual situation and to learn to recognise the problems in it and the methods of dealing with them. Being lectured to about problems and methods can help but can never take the place of direct experience.[1]

A further reason for the failure of the traditional courses is that they have not taken into consideration the fact that *the acquisition of psychotherapeutic skill does not consist only of learning something new: it inevitably also entails a limited, though considerable, change in the doctor's personality.*

### Clinical vignette

I will leave the scene to a group of general practitioners (GPs), whom I have been supervising during several years.

The session started with Clara almost bursting into a story about difficulties in handling a nurse at the clinic, continuing a story that goes on over years. This time the group became more engaged, listened and tried to relate to the difficulties of the presenter. Helen gave a detailed account from a parallel dilemma in her clinic and how it was solved. In the end Terry said: "We offer you all sorts of empathy, reflections and solutions; but you want none of it. I don't understand why you want to change the nurse?" Clara: "It is something inside myself. I don't know what it is; but it is inside me."

During the following round I mentioned my wish to use the group for a clinical vignette for a paper. The group decided to go on with this immediately to be sure to have the time. This could be a result of a long relation and knowledge to my tendency to get lost in cases —and an unexpected possibility to relate to the conductor? Feeling the interest and attention from an otherwise quite remote and neutral psychiatrist?

I asked them: "Psychotherapeutic education contains [one's] own experience in group or training analysis, what do you think about that, how come and which meaning does it have for your functions as psychotherapist and/or as a doctor?"

Clara: "I have been in a group as part of my training as Group Analyst and after that I had a short individual therapy. It brought clarity to the non-verbal interactions between the patient and me and helped me to separate my own material from the patients."

*The therapy is lived forwards and is understood backwards (*paraphrasing Kierkegaard: *Life is lived forwards and understood backwards*).

Jeremy: "I have been in individual therapy for years. The meaning of resistance became evident. If anything happened during the weekend before I went to therapy, something in the family where I got upset, I knew that I had to tell the therapist about how childish and unreasonably I had behaved. It was shameful. You have to tell about the emotional experiences otherwise it is a waste."

Sigmund: "I had 3 years in a group 30 years ago. I became free and didn't have to involve my unconscious anger in all the contacts I had with patients." I asked if it was in the therapies or in all consultations. "In all the consultations. The anger disappeared - people who knew me from before couldn't recognise me. What had happened to the angry man? (thinking) It is to be able to contain the patients without making it private. I got engaged with my own early tragedy and finished it."

Clara: "About containing. You can feel the tragedy in the other, use yourself to feel the other and stop when you feel, that she can't take any more. Not only can I contain more, I can also feel when the patient can't contain more."

Sigmund: "You can bear to feel it, to be reconciled with your own less flattering sides."

Clara: "I am tuned in on registration, have a greater attention on myself."

Jeremy: "It's okay to wait, we are always waiting for what will show up. I did put my therapist off with a lot of talk, that's what the patients do as well. That's the way it is."

Terry: "I've not been in therapy; but in supervision for 30 years if that counts. It is about being able to see the feelings of the patient without mingling yourself into them. See them next to your own stuff. To have peace with yourself. Not have to … the need to insist on one's own personality is not as big."

Sigmund: "As with free floating attention and at the same time focus. It is here Kierkegaard says that it is necessary to have a poetical capacity. You know that it is there. To be able to bear that others are in the same way as you and be able to talk about it. (A small pause) And that they are in other ways and still talk about it. It is not so shameful to be the one you are."

Clara: "The humility in asking and listening to the other - and separate it from yourself."

Helen, who is the youngest member of the group, has nothing to add.

I summarise: "To meet the other in the other and not oneself in the other" (also paraphrasing Kierkegaard).

Sigmund goes on with a new case. It's a woman in her twenties, brought by her mother. Texted tattoos on both arms – S. has not asked for the meaning of the text. He feels locked, held at a distance by her anger and silent weeping; knowing that any attempt to console her will provoke a rejection. She doesn't have any words and he can't find them. During the supervision he changes from a position where he wants her to hulk and cry deep to a more curious, open listening position, where he also has to listen to his own feelings.

Clara brings a follow up. The patient has a relapse in drinking and has been dismissed to the hospital in a bad shape. Clara worries if she has made too confronting and hurtful interpretations? And if she had a project on behalf of the patient?

The last is Terry about a supervision group, where only 3 of 5 members were present after the vacation. What to do? Jeremy says 'I would say something about it; I do so at the beginning of a new group. That we need each other if this is going to be a well-functioning group.'

**The role of the conductor**

As you might already have noticed I've chosen the term 'conductor' instead of leader.

The skill of the trained group conductor is to create an atmosphere in the group in which training can take place. It means (according to Balint) listening in the same way as we want the doctor to listen to his patient, letting the group members discover for themselves, and by this learning from the other members of the group through social integration, mirroring, exchange and resonance. The group members can develop the acceptance and appreciation of different attitudes between them, and each member can find their own way to listen to the patients.

The role of the conductor is to set the boundaries for the group regarding time and place; perhaps also for the setting and the way the group session is structured, leaving space for the presentation and reflection in the group. How the material is worked on, stressing the informative, formative or transformative aspects.

Basically, to conduct is to create a safe space with enough predictability, to keep the timing, and to know 'how far is too far' when confronting the group members.

## The influence of the relationship

The relationship between the group members and the conductor develops over time. We all know the feeling of an old group, where you know the members, their cases and their individual difficulties – as the members know each other and as they know the conductor. There the conductor can feel like a member of the group; but still has a special position as the one who keeps the boundaries of the group.

What influence does it have on the group and the dynamics in the group when there is a shift in conductor – and does it matter if it is a newly established group or an on-going, long-term group?

First and foremost, it is the task of the group conductor to keep the group in mind, which I think is also part of setting the frame. To listen to and pay attention to the group mind. How are the interactions in the group, the transferences, projections and identifications? Which role does the group member take or fall into again and again? To pay attention to avoid scapegoating and other malignant group processes.

Here the conductor's countertransference as it can be illustrated by the role of the group in the conductor's mind is crucial.

What meaning does it have that in a Balint Group the focus is on the doctor-patient relationship and especially on the illness influencing this? How does the illness influence the group, in another way than if it is a therapeutic group, and the relation is to family/spouse, or if it is a Balint Group for doctors?

## About starting a group – the first session and before

It is a special situation to collect a new group and to have it develop into a stable containing working-group relationship. Not to mention how to continue and let the group develop further over the years letting valuable members leave and new members come in and take their own seats.

## What did I learn at school?

I was trained as a Group Analyst in Aarhus in the early 1990s. It was the first year run by ourselves—the teachers from Aarhus with external supervision—in a flat structure that is still working. The supervisor shifts every 3rd year and in that way brings in new international inspiration and continuous education for the staff group.

Co-conducting the new Group was mandatory for us. It meant that I got a partner with whom I could discuss all my insecurity, questions, wishes, and dreams about the Group. It was part of the training to trust each other – and the group – enough to share our thoughts and reflections openly in the group and in that way, to become more aware of ourselves, the co-conductor, and the group. And I got a friend for life, with whom I'm still sharing dreams in a group.

During our training we used supervision hours to present assessments. Some of the then-young teachers got a publication that still can be traced in the paper by Kristian Valbak in 2018[2]. He concludes:

> For a group, take the patients who have a desire and are willing. Take the patients you can relate to in the assessment interview and whose problems you can empathize with. Do not rush through the assessment interview. What you have learned here will bless you later. Your preparation and that of the patient are the foundation for a successful group process, and the patients can learn for life from the assessment interview—even if they are not taken into therapy.[2]

### My present groups

I had the chance to start a psychotherapy group from zero some years ago. Five members were starting, one more came after half a year, and the last one after about a year. Two years into the group I had the feeling that the group had become more stable, the members attended the meetings regularly, almost on time, and they left apologies when not present. The first summer, after half a year, I announced my upcoming vacation for four or five weeks. Now I think it was far too early and too long a vacation, and I think it did contribute to my feeling of lack of coherence in the group.

The other side of the coin is that I need time to feel at home in a group; it takes time for the Matrix to develop. I wonder if next time I will plan for a more intensive start as a sort of block, meeting twice a day or twice a week during the introductory phase of the group.

These days I have a group that I have inherited from an elderly colleague, which means that there were six members in the group when I started as conductor—one of them is still there, one has come back for more treatment and is now staying for a longer period – and new members have arrived and concluded their treatment in the group. Some of them I still follow as their psychiatrist. The former group therapist takes over as substitute, when I'm away for instance for a conference, and the group feels confident and safe with her as I do. And furthermore, I have someone to exchange with about the group.

I think it is beneficial that the other conductor and I are trained in the same institute, we have the same profession and almost the same age (compared to the group members) and in that way share our foundation and social matrix to a certain degree. The Matrix of the group changes over time.

## A supervision group

I was asked to supervise a group of quite experienced group therapists as part of their training as group analysts, which has shown not to be much different from the training seminars we run for leadership training in Denmark.

After our initial meeting one of the members asked some very precise, simple and everlasting questions. They became the basis for many interesting and educational reflections in the group. She asked: "How many patients do we need in a group? I, for the moment, have three that I would like to form a group, I think that they could benefit from group therapy; but how many do I need to start? And where do I find them?"

Then the next question was, "What is the maximum number of members in the group?" The discussion crystalised around: "How does the conductor feel at ease in a group, in a new group, and in a well-known group?"

The group used an hour to discuss and reflect about the differences among themselves as conductors, how many members they feel at ease with, and what it means if there are too many members in the group. Will some stay away and will that be a relief for the group conductor, that the group is big enough to function with absences? Or is it more a question of how to establish a continuity and a feeling of belonging inside the group and between the group members, so they feel entitled to participate and be present? As my first supervisor used to say: [as a leader], the only reason for an absence is a funeral – one's own.

In the supervision group we also talked about how to conduct the first interview with a patient who seeks therapy and how to evaluate whether to offer group therapy. It's good to listen to the patient's former experiences in groups, their role in the family, at work, in sports, as scouts and in other social activities during life. For me it is useful to ask about siblings and their relationships and to try to get a feeling of any experiences of being scapegoated during school years or later. Such a process can help prevent dropout. A talk like that could also be adapted as part of the introductory process to a Balint Group for a doctor who expresses interest in joining.

Then there was the question about members from a former group who were not used to working in a group analytic way. "Is it possible to transfer one group into another format?," the question sounded. I think this is a very interesting, intriguing, and important question because it raises the question, what is real group analysis? Or what is a real Balint group? When have we found the Holy Grail, are we able to grab it and bring it with us into the group? What are the requirements, is it when we follow the rules and have strict frames or is it when we can be present in the group, with the group, as with ourselves as experienced or not-so- experienced group leaders.

Implied in these themes, as you will know, are the questions of how we want the group to function and what is the purpose of the group for the members and for the group leader?

We also had the question of payment of the leader, which is necessary to consider before starting the group. Generally, I find it positive for the alliance that the patient contributes in some way and there should be no question that I'm paid for my work as Group Analyst. The same is the case for my function in a Balint Group or as a supervisor.

## My group-analysis and Balint group

So here I come to the conscious and the unconscious mind of the conductor, that is, how we are feeling, thinking, and relating to ourselves and to the group, outside the group and in the group. We are affected by our preliminary fantasies, wishes and fears when we select members for the group, when we introduce the group to new members before they meet, and when the group meets.

I find it of importance to try to prevent drop-out, perhaps most critical when a new group is forming. One way to view this process is for all participants to find someone to identify with and for the group to contain the complexity of the society. It means that no one should be one-of-a-kind, meaning that I prefer to have more people who are the only child, both men and women, preferable with different sexual orientations. When holding groups in international settings, there are often different religious beliefs and nationalities among the group members. And they often have traumatic experiences in their family histories. I find it very stimulating to be allowed to work with this complexity of experience, traumas, and conflicts, and with the willingness to explore new land inside oneself and in the group.

Saying all this I have one group that is quite homogeneous because the one criterion for entering is to be a medical doctor. Despite that, it has functioned well over the years and offer long therapies for the members, who benefit from and appreciate the group.

The first years as group analyst I found myself (a bit) obsessive about the place, the arrangement of the chairs, the question of who unintendedly would/could walk into the group room while I was holding the group. Now I'm more observant of group members' different needs for comfortable chairs and interested in how they find their own place in the group. Generally, I want to introduce a new member or start a new group well ahead of any vacation and I try to announce vacations as early as possible. I no longer find any reason to frustrate the group intendedly, as it will happen anyway during the group.

For me, to be true to my inner group analyst is when I'm able to use my senses – my bodily feelings my associations, and my thinking capacity—to be present and to follow the movements in the group, listen to the pauses and the solos, and to intervene when I feel that the group in some way is out of tune.

I try to stimulate dream-telling by repeating the dream, ask the dreamer to repeat or the group to retell the dream. When working on the dream I try to redirect the comments from the group members to reflection on their own inner life by saying 'Try to make it your own dream', 'Try to say I', 'What would it be like if it was you, who dreamt like that?'. It's also a training and reminder for the group members to reflect on their own thoughts and prevent too many projections, labelling, and intellectualisation.

When is the group conceived? Is there an 'Annunciation Day' as Mary had with the Angel Gabriel appearing to her while she was reading and talking about her coming son, Jesus? For how long does the thought and wish for a group grow in the mind and body of the conductor, which dreams and wishes should be conscious, and how long should the gestation be, before the group can grow mature in the mind of the conductor and in reality?

In the leadership conferences we set ourselves a challenge by the structure to study and perhaps clarify the developing relationship between group and conductor. How are the group dynamics influenced by the continuity contrary to the shift in leadership?

If I've raised more questions than answers, that was my purpose.

The first words and the instruction for the group is important in any group. The formulation might be dependent on whether it's a new group or has met before and developed its matrix; but still there are new members and in that way it becomes a new group.

I would like to say welcome to all of you in this large group. I have now been the presenter in the group. The group gives us the opportunity to share our thoughts, feelings, dreams and whatever comes to our minds. Remember about confidentiality: that what is said in the group stays in the group.

I think it's very important to be able to speak up about our fears and try to loosen the anxiety to make the communication and the dialogue freer, more open end rewarding for the group members. Everyone is free to speak up. Please, let the conference begin.

Tove Mathiesen, MD
Group Analyst, Psychoanalyst (IPA), Psychiatrist
President, International Balint Federation

References:
Balint, M. *The doctor, the patient and the illness.* p. 299

Valbak K. Preparing for group analytic psychotherapy: meeting the new patient. Group Analysis 2018;51:159-74.

Thanks to Guang Yu for his inspiration that led to some of these thoughts.

# Ascona Prize Essays

The Ascona Prize is granted by the Psychosomatic and Social Medicine Foundation for medical students from all countries. €5,000 is available for the authors of the three best essays. The articles are in English.

The essay must describe a student-patient relationship, a personal experience from the student's medical studies, a description of how they lived this relationship, the way they responded to it, and finally a critical reflection on the evolution of their state of consciousness and the way to improve it.

# 1. Ausweingärtner[1]

Julian Neugebauer

University of Muenster – School of Medicine
Germany

It is 2:30 p.m. on Friday afternoon. Despite a low turnover on the psychiatric ward, the morning had been exhausting due to spontaneous discharges and a staffing level decimated by COVID infections. I was just looking forward to the upcoming weekend when I received the news that there had been another new admission. Equipped with a laptop for documentation, I accompany the senior physician to the admission interview in our ward room. On the way there, we are briefly informed by the attentive nursing staff that the patient is a medical colleague. When we enter the room, we are greeted in a friendly and direct manner by an obviously hyperactive woman in her fifties, who, when I introduce myself as a PJ student, promptly replies: "Now listen carefully, you could write your doctoral thesis about me!"

## 1. Exposition
### The first impression
When I met Ms. K. for the first time on that Friday, I had no idea that she would be right in part and that she would trigger so many impulses in me.

At the beginning of the intake interview, everything seemed routine. Mrs. K. had been suffering from Parkinson's disease for years and her medication could explain her hypermotoric. She had also undergone a bilateral mastectomy two weeks ago. She described that a few days ago she was violently attacked by her neighbor, who hit her on the wound on her chest in the stairwell. In addition, something that could be detected by magnetic radiation had been implanted during the mastectomy. Her great fear of being followed by the neighbor was evident in every sentence and she repeated several times that she did not think she would survive the night.

Her eagerness to talk coupled with her technical eloquence made the conversation really special. She was always friendly, but showed no insight into her illness and, due to her background knowledge, often found a way to challenge our arguments with an inconceivable, minimal residual probability of the opposite. As we were firmly convinced that we could help her well with this symptomatology, but there was no basis for forcing her into treatment, we aimed to convince her to stay voluntarily. After almost two and a half hours, during which the senior physician conducted the conversation with the patience of a saint, we finally succeeded in persuading Ms. K. to stay in hospital voluntarily.

Somewhat exhausted, I collected my things after the interview and was about to leave for the weekend when Mrs. K. asked me to sit on a bench next to her because she wanted to show me something. I set up internet access on her tablet and she tried to download an app for detecting magnetic radiation. The download process stopped several times, so she decided to tell me why. She knew that her fellow patients had jammers in their cigarette packs that would connect to the part in her chest and cause her terrible pain.

After this, I was finally sure that she was in good hands on the ward. I left the clinic with the good feeling of knowing that Mrs. K. was now being treated and with the firm expectation that in her case, for once, the symptoms could be alleviated relatively "quickly and sustainably".

When I returned to work on Monday morning, I found out that Mrs. K. had discharged herself a few hours later against medical advice. This depressed me a little, as not only did all the effort seem to have been in vain, but I was also firmly convinced that we could have helped Mrs. K. quickly with good medication. But if there was one thing I had already learned, it was that you usually see each other more than once in a lifetime in psychiatry...

**The reunion**
It happened as expected and a week later Mrs. K. was transferred back to us from another psychiatric ward by PsychKG[2]. We found out that she had actually been beaten by her neighbor and had broken two ribs. However, the imaging of her head carried out in a somatic emergency room after this incident was unremarkable. In addition, her breast had become inflamed in the meantime, so that accompanying gynecological treatment had to be sought. All these somatic ailments, which could now be objectified, apparently reinforced Ms. K.'s impression that she had no psychological component. At the same time, this made it difficult for us to convince Ms. K. of the need for drug therapy for her psychological symptoms. She only took some of the prescribed medication and refused to take an antipsychotic. The PsychKG in particular was an enormous burden for Ms. K., as she felt "locked in" and was not used to having to relinquish control in her life. The whole team had numerous conversations with her, reassured her and waited for a change.

**Cloud 7**
After another week, it became apparent that Mrs. K. was becoming increasingly more orderly in thinking. Although she was still refusing to take antipsychotics, she had gained the trust of the ward doctor with neurological experience, who optimized her Parkinson's medication and explained to her in detail the reasons for each individual dosage.

During a visit, she recited a poem she had written herself ("7 strong clouds") and told us that we had animals in the walls. Ms. K. suggested "objectifying" this with a simple experiment so that she could show that she wasn't crazy and we could finally lift the PsychKG. Contrary to my expectations, the experienced senior physician agreed to this "experiment". So we went into Mrs. K's room and watched as she began to remove the plaster from the wall with a fork. When nothing could be seen at the first spot, Mrs. K. changed the spot again and began to pick at another side of the wall with the fork. Nothing was visible here either. Ms. K. then got her SLR camera and tried to photograph the lamps in the room so that the animals hiding there could be seen. But none of the photos produced the desired result. Somewhat disappointed, she realized that we had apparently been right.

Since the "experiment", Ms. K. seemed to have gained even more trust in us. Two days later, we were even able to lift the PsychKG prematurely, as she was able to give us credible assurances that she would remain in treatment voluntarily. She even started taking the antipsychotic medication "on a trial basis" soon afterwards.

One morning when I had just arrived on the ward, she was waiting for me at the entrance and pressed her poem "7 Strong Clouds" into my hand. It was a gift for me, she said. Because I would have known which cloud was her "Ausweingarten". I had already been touched by the beautiful poem during the visit, but the fact that she even gave it to me was a special honor and joy!

### 7 Starke Wolken
*Wenn eine eiskalte Hand dein Herz in Schutt + Asche legt,*
*und niemand mit dir fühlt, was es so fehl-erregt,*
*dann lehrt es dich durch's einsam überleben,*
*daß in all den schönen Zwischenräumen*
*zwischen Himmel, Erde, Bäumen*
*in reichlich Platz aus Lust am Leben,*
*7 starke Wolken kleben.*

*Die 1. ist zum Ordnen.*
*Die 2. zum Korrigieren.*
*Die 3. die kann tragen,*
*die 4. kann man alles fragen,*
*die 5. hat `nen Ausweingarten,*
*die 6. läßt fließen*
*+ dann kommt Wolke 7*
*zum Lieben*

*(Für meine geduldigen Ärzte mit Team, die mit mir sämtliche Wolken durchmachten, damit meine 7 bleibt)*

*7 strong clouds*

*If no one feels with you what makes it so wrong,*
*then it teaches you to survive through loneliness,*
*that in all the beautiful spaces*
*between sky, earth, trees*
*in abundant space for the pleasure of living,*
*7 strong clouds cling.*

*The 1st is for organizing.*
*The 2nd is for correcting.*
*The 3rd can carry,*
*the 4th can be asked anything,*
*the 5th has a Ausweingarten,*
*the 6th lets flow*
*+ then comes cloud 7*
*to love*

*(For my patient doctors and team who went through all the clouds with me so that my 7 stays)*

## 2. Reflection

### Treatment relationship with Mrs. K. - Poetry makes medicine

The poem triggered in me an intensive reflection on the treatment relationship with Mrs. K., which was not primarily rational, but rather characterized by emotional understanding through the poetry. For this reason, I would like to use the structure of the poem as a guide when writing down my reflections.

### 1st cloud – organizing

Like Ms. K., many patients are not sorted at the beginning of their stay in psychiatry. As a term used in psychopathological assessment, I had therefore been quite familiar with this term. However, its positioning as the first cloud of the poem made it clear to me that this is not a mere symptom description, but an important and elementary step in the recovery process. Of course, I remember some situations in which things got out of hand and I needed time and peace to collect myself. However, I can in no way measure how intense the feeling of inner chaos must be when you not only lose control and confidence in your perception, but are also forced into a completely unknown environment by a decision of the state authorities. This verse by Ms. K. made her intense fear and mistrust really tangible for me for the first time. In such a situation, sorting things out could only happen within herself and could not be forced from outside. She needed time and the treatment team needed patience. For me, this patience is the central element from which all the clouds, the metaphor for her steps in the recovery process, are woven. Contrary to my impressive experience of an always tight clinical time corset in most internships during my studies, it was a really profound experience for me to have to give Mrs. K. the necessary time to start a recovery process and to be able to do this increasingly better.

## 2nd cloud – correcting

In contrast to somatic disciplines such as surgery or internal medicine, where the cause of the illness is treated "from the outside" by the practitioner through targeted intervention, I believe that mental illnesses require a great deal of active processing by the patient. The patient is not primarily - as I have often encountered in clinical traineeships - a passive object in which a broken bone is set or an electrolyte imbalance is rebalanced with medication, but as the main actor must muster the strength to independently integrate the impulses set by the environment into the world view. In order for this correction to be successful, I believe that not only an orderly state of consciousness is required, but in particular the presentation of offers tailored to the individual. Of course, medication can be one such group of offers, but its strengths seem to me to lie primarily in symptom management.

In the case of Ms. K., the right offer was the experiment described in the exposition. How often was I present or active myself when we tried to influence Mrs. K. in long arguments? But it was only the patient offer of the senior physician, which gave Mrs. K. the freedom to convince herself of the hallucination, that brought about a change in her world view. I personally think that Mrs. K.'s need to be convinced through self-awareness was due to her fear, which was fed by the feeling of loss of control. This insight was of immense importance for the further treatment, as we now knew better which offers we could suggest to Mrs. K.. In a similar manner, I was allowed to accompany her to an appointment with the head physician of the breast center where the mastectomy was performed. As the head physician took a lot of time to answer Mrs. K's questions in detail, I felt that I had a lot of time too. I could literally see with every minute how the inner tension that had been building up in Mrs. K. for days was easing.

Impressed by the sustainability of these treatments, my understanding of the role of a medical student or doctor changed. What I thought of as holistic medicine was subject to a point of view error. For me, it previously meant looking at as many areas of a person as possible and developing the most optimal pathogenetic-oriented intervention from this, but always from a perspective where I was the actor, the "problem solver". The treatment relationship with Ms. K. broadened my perspective and showed me that it is more productive - especially in the case of mental illness - to be a companion who offers connectable support - often also as a "Ausweingärtner".

## 3rd cloud – carrying

For a correction to be sustainable, it seems important to me that a fragile change in the world view of the person undergoing treatment is supported by the environment. He or she must experience that the correction is sustainable and reliable. When Ms. K. once saw animals in her room lamps, we tried to capture them with her SLR camera. No matter from which perspective we photographed, the pictures always showed ordinary lampshades. This not only led to Mrs. K. being able to distance herself more and more from such perceptions, but in my view also strengthened the treatment relationship enormously by "experimenting" together. Mrs. K. built up more and more trust in the ward doctor and me. This trust was incredibly valuable, as it gave us the opportunity, for example, to convincingly supplement the personal support offered with medication. While I had previously believed in the Habermasian coercion of the better argument when giving medication, Mrs. K. taught me to appreciate the non-coercive advice of a confidant.

### 4th cloud – asking

If you have a lot of (specialist) knowledge like Ms. K., there are all the more points of contact for uncertainties, so I could empathize with her great urge to ask questions. I remember too well the phase during my studies when, after reading almost every clinical picture, I thought that the symptoms actually applied to me too. After a while, however, the habituation effects were so strong that I switched to the opposite and ignored my own body signals in a feeling of inviolability until I finally had to go to the clinic as a patient with a serious illness myself. I had a déjà vu with Mrs. K. and saw myself again in the same clinic, where my dangerous half-knowledge constantly fueled my fear and I inwardly doubted every treatment approach because there was still a study there that did it differently or the pharmacology slide said that you just shouldn't take a certain combination of drugs. For this reason, I was able to empathize with Mrs. K. particularly well. It was easy for me to answer her numerous questions with patience and to the best of my knowledge, as I was well aware of the great reassurance potential that answers and empathy can bring.

In the course of reflection, I then asked myself whether I show the same level of commitment to others, even though I sometimes find it more difficult to emotionally relate to them. Unfortunately, the answer is quite clear, as I invested significantly more time than usual in the relationship work with Mrs. K.. Just because other patients don't demand as much time and perhaps can't formulate as many questions doesn't mean that their illness is any less complex, let alone less painful. I would therefore like to take away from Cloud 4 that there are many sufferers who are unable to express their inner fears and tensions in any questions or words and that this should not be a reason to assume that they are absent.

### 5th cloud – "Ausweingarten"

Mrs. K. was particularly proud of this cloud. For me, the neologism of the "Ausweingarten" stands for a place where you feel safe and protected and where you can sort out your thoughts. For me, this atmosphere of trust and security is the prerequisite for being able to cry at all. Linking this place with the idea of a garden really appeals to me. I am a person who feels a great sense of connection and peace in nature. For example, when I go mountain climbing, I feel very humble before the vastness of nature and feel part of a larger whole. This often leads to my own problems and needs fading into the background in these moments, sometimes even seeming very small and unimportant. Combining this feeling of nature with a place to cry and creating such a space in the clinic seems to me to be a very noble goal.

I also find the metaphor very successful because the elixir of a magnificent garden is not expensive gold, but water. Perhaps even the very water that is released when we cry. This interpretation applies well to Mrs. K., because in my opinion, she drew the strength from crying to be able to stand up again.

### 6th cloud – Flow

For me, flow has something dynamic about it and goes in a certain direction. For this reason, the 6 cloud can be understood as the actual (minimum) goal in the recovery process. For me, this is where the rigidity and constriction during an illness is dissolved.

In relation to Mrs. K., this cloud also has an intensely physical component. She suffered not only from hyper-, but also from hypomotor phases as part of her Parkinson's disease. I find it hard to imagine the feeling of being trapped in one's own body. It is perhaps most comparable to the sleep paralysis I experienced some time ago. I can still feel the fear from back then, but my immobility was in a dream world in my head. In Mrs. K.'s case, this helplessness existed within interpersonal interaction. It is understandable to me that she was incompliant with such a wealth of experience and preferred not to take too much medication in order to get into the hypermotoric phase. The sensitive approach of the ward doctor, who determined the medication together with Mrs. K. almost every day and in this way guided her step by step into the optimal setting, seemed all the more exemplary to me.

### Cloud 7 – Love

For me, loving means being able to do something for someone else. However, when you are ill, you have to concentrate on yourself and focus all your energy on recovery. Helping a person to regain so much strength that they can not only give something back to themselves, but also to someone else, i.e. to be able to love, is the most beautiful goal of treatment for me.

In psychiatry in particular, the environment is closely linked to the patient's situation, so the treatment work often has a far-reaching effect on an entire social structure. The treatment relationship with Mrs. K. made this very clear to me. Her husband suffered greatly from seeing his wife in this state. At the beginning of her treatment, Mrs. K. was very suspicious of him and often accused him of not supporting her properly. When her condition gradually improved, a few days after she had presented her poem to us on the ward round, she came back from a walk around town with her husband wearing a beautiful new necklace around her neck. The necklace was adorned with a large, blue, drop-shaped gemstone set in silver, which drew the eye to her breastbone. She told me that it was a gift from her husband, who normally didn't buy her such expensive things on the spur of the moment. For her, this necklace is now a symbolic "declaration of war" against all the things that have happened to her since her mastectomy. Now she wants to tackle them. Whenever I met her in the corridor in the days that followed, she would simply tap the necklace with her index finger and I noticed how a broad smile always spread beneath my mask.

To be seen as someone who has made a small contribution to her being able to love again by dedicating her poem flatters me and makes me very happy!

### The team – all for one
In my clinic, I was lucky enough to work in an interdisciplinary and multi-professional treatment team that managed to work together as equals.

This credit goes above all to the senior physician and the nursing management, who created an atmosphere in which everyone was able to contribute their skills and was appreciated for it. In Mrs. Ks. poem, this treatment environment is well reflected in the image of the "Ausweingarten", because if you see the patients as plants in this garden, it takes more than just a gardener to make the flowers grow again. Social services could provide sunshine, medicine could fertilize the soil, psychology could provide a supporting skeleton, nursing could water, etc.

Nevertheless, I know that this kind of collaboration requires a great deal of effort to structure and organize. Being part of the many meetings - with their different compositions - and experiencing the enormous communication skills required for such a round of talks made a lasting impression on me. I have a vivid memory of how the senior physician once put her point of view aside and decided against her own position in favor of the majority opinion, even though she was the one who was solely responsible.

I could literally feel how I had arrived in the team after a while, when I was able to make my first contributions and contribute my student perspective. Thanks to my good treatment relationship with Ms. K., I was not only listened to, but was also able to use this to help the others in the treatment team better understand Ms. K's actions.

The relationship with my ward doctor was also particularly formative for me. We shared responsibility for Mrs. K's case and I enjoyed the luxury of being able to invest a lot of time in a complex case like Mrs. K's in psychiatry. We had long discussions, pored over the literature to better narrow down a possible etiology and developed treatment ideas, as we had learned from Mrs. K's "experiment" that an experiential approach could be very effective for her. Thanks to the constant exchange and direct feedback on my ideas, Mrs. K's treatment was very exciting and productive for me. It was not uncommon for questions to arise from our conversation that touched on my own ethical ideas. Suddenly it wasn't just about Mrs. K., but about a general understanding of how you want to fulfill your role as a doctor. The critical openness and willingness of the ward doctor to discuss this not only on an abstract level, but also to incorporate his feelings and experiences from his clinical work, gave me a lot of food for thought. Once when we were discussing the thresholds of a possible forced medication of Mrs. K., I was impressed by his tireless optimism that Mrs. K. would take her medication voluntarily. Based on this conviction, he initially stopped the Parkinson's medication for over a week, in daily consultation with Mrs. K, until she had gained enough trust in him to voluntarily try taking another antipsychotic. I was very impressed by his willingness to choose the ethical path over the more comfortable one - despite the great effort and rather low chances of success - and to draw so much patience from this.

## 3. Action

While I had been thinking about Mrs. K.'s poem for a few days, I discovered a reminder of the Balint-Prize in my mailbox. The first sentence that Mrs. K. had said to me immediately came to mind. As many threads of thought were still buzzing around in my head and I was still very moved by the poem, I plucked up my courage and described to Ms. K. my idea of writing down our treatment relationship pseudonymously and submitting it. I was surprised that she not only immediately gave her consent, but was also immensely happy about it. We then talked at length about my interpretation of her poem and the lessons I had learned from it. Two major goals emerged for me: to become more patient in treatment relationships and to pay more attention to people who are less able to articulate their fears and needs.

### Patience

Ms. K. confirmed to me several times how important the patience shown by the treatment team had been for her. In a situation in which she was largely deprived of her freedom, at least allowing her the autonomy to make her own decisions about her medication was a very important support. I would also like to try to provide this support in the future and support such experiences of self-efficacy.

In two months' time, I'll be moving on to my surgery tertial. The high time pressure there seems to me to be an ideal testing ground for practising patience under systemic pressure. Of course, I realize that I will encounter different time corridors there than in psychiatry, but I believe that a patient attitude can be felt quickly in the high-frequency, somatic hospital routine, even on a small scale. Whether it's in the information session, where I try to ask questions to make sure that the procedure has really been understood, or in the emergency room, where I don't want to interrupt the first answer after 10 seconds, but want to leave time to tell the story. Particularly when it comes to prescribing medication, I see great potential for increasing compliance through patient education. I have the feeling that due to the unanimous professional evidence - e.g. for some long-term medications - there is often little empathy on the part of doctors for those being treated, or at least this is not expressed due to the performance-oriented time pressure. This is why, in my opinion, patients are given (too) little time to accept the need for medication and thus convince themselves of its relevance. I would like to counter this form of persuasive education with patient persuasion and learn to endure the fact that medically indicated therapy proposals can also be rejected (for the time being). For me, this also implies being open to unusual treatment methods in further training in order to have more individually tailored treatment suggestions in my repertoire and to be able to offer them as an alternative.

### Quiet waters

When writing down the reflection, I realized that I am very involved in treatment relationships in which a lot is demanded of me. However, those who do not express their fears and are perhaps not even aware of their needs are neglected. In future, I would like to be more proactive in my approach to these patients and take them into consideration. In concrete terms, this means that I want to take the time to put myself in the other person's shoes in every treatment relationship and find out what emotions are currently guiding their actions.

This was very easy for me with Ms. K., but when I subsequently tried to do the same with more reserved people, I noticed how difficult it could be to grasp the individual emotional state. Although I had diligently given items in the psychopathological assessment that described the affect in a structured way, I could not say why someone was depressed or what the hopelessness arose from. For this reason, a huge range of connecting factors remained closed to me in these treatment relationships.

## 4. Progression
### Disturbances have priority
Ruth Cohn's postulate "Disturbances have priority!" from Theme-Centered Interaction (TCI) seems to me to be very important for responsible medical action. It can be easily adapted to treatments, as the disorders are often not at the content level but at the relationship level. In everyday clinical practice, the focus is usually on the professional dimension and the relationship level is minimized through distanced behaviour in the understanding of professionalization. Especially with people like Ms. K., this seems fatal to me, as the relationship level is a necessary condition for a substantive discussion. In my opinion, it would be desirable to adopt more perspectives in both medical and student activities in order to include the relationship level more strongly.

For me, empathizing with another perspective begins with the common use of statements in doctors' letters such as "The patient introduced himself..." , "The patient reports ..." "The patient was ... under treatment" or "We recommend the patient ...". These phrases seem disrespectful to me. From my point of view, they do not express the necessary appreciation for another person who has a name and a story. I think such formulations contribute to reification, which is also emphasized on the ward when a distinction is made between "room 266 window or door". In the end, this reification culminates in the allocation according to certain disease categories, when only "the gall bladder", "the liver" or "the appendix" are mentioned.

I would like every practitioner to regularly try to empathize with the patient's perspective before making a decision and to critically reflect on their own position in this regard. Simple questions such as "How do you feel when you meet Mrs. Müller?", "How does it feel to be on dialysis for years like Mr. Müller?", "How do you feel when you think about Mrs. Müller's future?" can be used to get a sense of the emotional situation. This complements the purely functional dimension, as you are involved in the treatment relationship as a person who is capable of feeling. Just as it is routine to inquire about certain areas in the medical history, such questions should be an integral part of a treatment routine.

## Persuasion medicine

Reflecting on the clouds from Mrs. K's poem made me realize that the doctor's role includes both the active problem solver and the supportive companion. Here I see a connection to argumentation theory, where the distinction between persuasion and convincing has existed since antiquity. While persuasion is done with manipulative intent, persuasion aims to persuade an individual to adopt an attitude to action by means of testimony. The similarity lies in the perspective. Just as the listener is the decisive subject in argumentation, who convinces himself of something and is not convinced, it is the treated person in (psychological) medicine who is not talked into recovery, but heals himself through support that can be connected.[3]

For me, this means that medical practice needs to be aware of this dual role of problem solver and companion, even in specialties that are not oriented towards conversational medicine. Because as soon as a somatic illness is coupled with a stressful, psychological component, such as in the case of tumors or chronic illnesses, both roles are needed for the recovery process. For training and further education, I would therefore like to see more training on when the focus should be on active (problem) solving and when we should see ourselves more as companions who provide individuals with resources that promote their health and well-being.

## Structures

Based on the realization of the great potential that can be found in involving oneself with one's feelings in a treatment relationship and the awareness of having to meet the requirements of both a problem solver and an accompanying insight helper, I believe that new spaces for this emotional reflection are needed in everyday clinical practice. Of course, some of these spaces already exist (Balint groups etc.), but the decisive criterion for me would be integration into the daily work routine. Just as a physical and psychopathological examination of the patient is part of the standard toolkit, a kind of mini-emotional status of the practitioner seems to me to be an enrichment in order to professionalize a more empathic attitude in the treatment relationship.

I am very surprised that there are a number of AMWF guidelines, but not a single one that deals with the culture of communication in medicine across disciplines. As deeply differentiated as the professional content level is in evidence-based medicine, the relationship level in medical contexts seems to be superficially illuminated. For me, efforts are therefore needed to establish evaluable communication structures in order to create resonance spaces for empathy and joint reflection and ultimately make communication in treatment relationships more successful in this way.

The entire reflection on and with Ms. K. convinced me that it is personally beneficial for me to integrate a mini-emotional state into my routines. The experience of how my own emotions brought into the treatment relationship can enrich it has permanently changed my whole attitude with which I now enter into further treatment relationships.

My challenge now is to translate these insights into appropriate attitudes and actions on a daily basis.

## Epilogue

I read this report together with Mrs. K. on the day it was handed in. It may not have become a doctoral thesis, but it worked on my understanding of "being a doctor". Wrestling with certain formulations in the writing process brought me to a level of reflection that I would not have reached through purely cognitive analysis. However, being able to reflect not only on my own or as part of the treatment team, but also to engage in a metacommunicative exchange with Ms. K. about the patient's perspective, was a formative experience that had a lasting effect and for which I am very grateful to her! We found a common projection surface in the "Ausweingarten". Here, Mrs. K. was able to forget her worldly worries, gather strength and feel free. Similar to the biblical Garden of Eden, the "Ausweingarten" is a paradisiacal, utopian place of refuge for Mrs. K.. By allowing me to go with her to this place, I was able to support her in a different way than in the usual role relationship of a treatment relationship. This form has lasted far beyond the initial meeting and has formed the basis of our contact ever since. Using the power of metaphors, both Ms. K. and I were able to express our respective feelings, make them understandable to the other person and thus become effective. As an example, I would like to mention the fantastic idea of the "Seelenkompost"[4]. After Ms. K. had shown this text to her family and friends, we received initial feedback and tried to process it together. As expected, the "Ausweingarten" triggered the most response, so we reflected on the impulses. Suddenly Mrs. K. said that for her, it was not the cross-references to the Garden of Eden, Adam and Eve or a painted paradise that were in the foreground, but the small riches of the garden, such as a "Seelenkompost". This is a source of new growth for those who have enough patience to nurture and care for the garden. Here, what had once blossomed and then withered could become something new. The whole wealth of different life events, which are presented in the numerous plants in the garden, could blossom anew with a little (gardening) work and time on the "Seelenkompost". In addition, sometimes a good digging is needed to keep the compost fertile.

This metaphor describes our treatment relationship so impressively and wonderfully, and has since then influenced me to use the power of figurative language. Thanks to Mrs. K., I often think of the 7 clouds of the poem in difficult moments with patients, especially of the "Ausweingarten" and the "Seelenkompost". They remind me that sometimes a patient gardener is needed to help with the "Seelenkompost". But also how arduous and persistent it is to try to be one every day.

**Footnotes**

[1] "Ausweingärtner" is a German neologism derived from the treatment relationship described here. It refers to a gardener in a very special garden, namely the "Ausweingarten". An "Ausweingarten" is a metaphorical word creation that plays with the homophony of crying and wine in German. On the one hand, the term creates the image of a beautiful vineyard and, on the other, of a place where you can cry out your sorrows. The term "Ausweingärtner" therefore refers to the ward doctor and me as a practitioner, as we supported Mrs. K. in her work in her "Ausweingarten".

[2] PsychKG is the common abbreviation for the Mental Illness Acts, i.e. German state laws that regulate the detention of mentally ill people in a specialist psychiatric hospital in the event of acute danger to themselves or others.

[3] In Socratic maieutics, this becomes particularly clear linguistically, as this technique literally means midwifery. The rhetorical insight helper and the midwife both have a supporting function in something that originally comes from itself.

[4] Another neologism that can be translated as soul compost.

# All the Good Things, but Solitude

Mateus Menezes

Federal University of São Paulo -- Paolista School of Medicine
Brazil

At the beginning of my second year of medical school, my desire for more opportunities for practical activities and the improvement of human skills led me to co-found an Academic League of Narrative Medicine, based on the principles of Rita Charon. The aim was clear: to establish a space for sincere dialog between students and patients. The conversation takes place at the university's pediatric infectious diseases clinic. Even before the patients were seen by the doctors, our meetings provided a unique opportunity to connect, far from the formality of a medical history. The professors in charge asked for the patients' permission beforehand, respecting their privacy and autonomy. In a private room, we students gave ourselves over to the art of empathetic listening, hoping to understand not only the clinical manifestations of diseases, but the human stories that surrounded them. After these conversations, we wrote chronicles or any other type of literary production about this meeting and then met as a group to discuss and share our experiences.

Longitudinal follow-up of children and adolescents who have contracted HIV through vertical transmission is very common in this clinic. One day, at one of these meetings organized by the Narrative Medicine Academic League, I was introduced to a mother who accompanied her son to all his appointments. I'll call them Eliza and Ruan, who was not in the room at the time of the conversation because only his mother agreed to take part. Eliza, a 55-year-old brown woman, wore a sad, worried expression, with a penetrating, frightened look that revealed the complexities of her journey as a caregiver for a son with HIV. Upon entering the room, the first observation that caught my attention was the fact that Eliza was wearing two N95 masks, even during a period of low COVID-19 contagion and with the boiling heat outside. This behavior clearly reveals her extreme concern not only for her own protection, but above all for the safety of her son.

***

As students in the first few years, we have more openness and time for more subjective and in-depth conversations about the non-physiological aspects that permeate patients' lives. However, when I observe older doctors and professors, I realize that this possibility disappears over time as we progress through the course. Medical practice, often shaped by logistical issues and high demand in the single health system, especially in a country of continental dimensions like Brazil, becomes marked by quick consultations focused exclusively on the pathophysiology of the disease. The need to attend to a large volume of patients often limits the depth of interactions, directing the focus towards adjusting drug doses and requesting complementary tests to ensure disease control.

This transition throughout the course highlights the challenges faced in managing the gap between paying attention to the patient's subjectivity and ensuring the efficiency needed to meet the demands of the health system. It is a reflection on how, as we move forward, medical practice can move away from the richness of narratives to the detriment of the flow of care.

There in the room, alone with the patient, I felt enormously responsible. It seemed that the environment transcended the physical space of a few square meters. Although I was aware that my role did not involve prescribing medication or making clinical decisions, the feeling of responsibility was gigantic. It was clear to me that, at that moment, I wasn't just a medical student; to her, I represented the institution and, in a way, a medical professional, albeit one in training. The loneliness shared in that space resonated with the patient's vulnerability. I was alone for the first time with a mother, a guardian who was deeply concerned about the health of the human being she loved most in the world: her son. Even though it was a follow-up appointment, I realized the immense emotional charge that permeated that encounter. At that moment, I viscerally understood the magnitude of the trust that patients place in their doctors.

The patient's vulnerability in front of us, students and health professionals, is a fine thread that connects medicine to the most human essence of existence. In these initial moments, the mother exposed her greatest fears and worries, confiding not only her clinical concerns, but also the emotions echoing in her chest because of her son's medical condition. This experience highlighted the delicacy of this relationship of trust between doctor and patient, showing that, in addition to technical knowledge, the ability to be compassionate and receptive to vulnerabilities is fundamental to truly humanized medical practice. After all, being vulnerable in front of another person is one of the most intrinsically human expressions and, at the same time, one of the most precious gifts that a patient can offer to those who are attending to them.

At the start of the conversation I wanted to understand everything from the beginning, so I asked Eliza how it all began, how she found out she was HIV positive and what it was like to deal with this reality. She shared an account full of emotions and marked by a series of impactful events. Eliza admitted that she wasn't sure how she contracted the virus, but suspected that it came from a blood transfusion she had to have around the age of 30.

Eliza shared with me her journey as a Jehovah's Witness, a faith that forbids blood transfusions. This restriction initially seemed to be an explanation for not revealing the real means by which she contracted the HIV virus. At a delicate moment in our conversation, I decided to ask her if the people in her religious community were aware of her transfusion, and Eliza, in a quick and visibly embarrassed gesture, confirmed it with her head. Later, when discussing it with my teachers, I realized that Eliza had mixed this transfusion narrative with the possibility of betrayal on the part of her partner at the time. The precise details of the infection remained unclear to us. I understood that my role at the time was not to uncover the intimate details of Eliza's life, especially when this information would not alter her condition that had already been established for years.

The complexity of Eliza's situation vividly illustrated the intersection between religious beliefs, personal relationships and health. As a medical student, I was confronted with the importance of understanding and respecting the diversity of patients' life experiences, recognizing that individual choices and beliefs can significantly influence health care decisions. The ethical dilemma that Eliza faced in relation to her faith and her health condition highlighted the complexities that healthcare professionals can encounter when dealing with religious issues. In a diverse society, where religious beliefs shape people's perspectives and decisions, it is crucial to approach these issues with sensitivity and respect. Throughout our conversation, I realized that Eliza was looking not just for a listener, but for someone who understood the multiplicity of challenges she faced. Her willingness to share her story indicated not only the need for medical support, but also for understanding and acceptance. Although the specific details of the infection remained inconclusive, the experience with Eliza highlighted the importance of a humanized approach in medical practice.

So I decided to continue the conversation respecting her space and prioritizing the information she felt comfortable sharing with me.

The starting point of this story, in her memory, was confused with the emotional news of the birth of her son and the simultaneous and overwhelming diagnosis that she was HIV positive. The moment she received the diagnosis was described by Eliza as a dry run. There was no preparation or any kind of welcome. The flood of information, added to the presence of her baby in her arms, left her dazed and with no prospects of seeking help immediately for her own treatment, she confesses. Apart from the fact that at the time, the therapeutic arsenal and prognosis were different, much more limited, the lack of support at this crucial moment deeply marked her initial experience with HIV. Eliza's story became even more distressing when, three and a half years into Ruan's life, she discovered that her son was also HIV positive. This revelation, according to her, is *"the greatest burden she will carry for as long as she lives."*

An overwhelming sense of guilt accompanies her, even though she knows that the bond between mother and child transcends any form of individual responsibility. This emotional weight has become a constant burden in her journey as a mother and caregiver.

Eliza became emotional as she told me this. This simple but deeply symbolic gesture encapsulated the pain and vulnerability that permeated her story. The tears, along with all the stigma presented by society, were silent expressions of a heavy emotional burden, a testimony to the strength and fragility present in Eliza and Ruan's lives. During our conversation, amid the sweltering 30°C heat in the stuffy room, the only thing that touched Eliza's mask were her tears. At that moment, I kept myself from bursting into tears with her.

The impactful story of how Eliza was diagnosed with a disease that would forever shape the course of her life led me to reflect deeply on the role we play as health professionals. It became clear to me the absurd influence we have on patients' lives. The way we handle the disclosure of sensitive information can cause significant consequences, leaving deep and lasting marks on their life experiences. That's why it was such a privilege just to be able to listen to what this woman had to say. At this point in our conversation, Eliza looked at me with eyes filled with feelings of guilt and anger at herself, but also with a certain relief at being able to share this very honest feeling with someone. It was at that moment that, for the first time during my medical course, I was able to internalize more deeply the meaning of Carl Jung's famous quote:

*"Know all the theories, master all the techniques, but when you touch a human soul, be just another human soul."*

This maxim transcended mere academic learning and came to life in Eliza's emotionally charged, stuffy room. By recognizing her vulnerability and allowing myself to be vulnerable as a listener, I discovered that our shared humanity is a powerful bridge in the doctor-patient relationship.

This episode reinforced the importance of cultivating empathy, recognizing the ethical responsibility we bear and understanding that behind every diagnosis there is a unique and delicate human story. I learned that medical practice goes beyond the application of technical knowledge; it's also about the art of caring, offering emotional support and recognizing the power of human connection in the healing journey.

The atmosphere in the room, now calmer, was charged with the words Eliza shared as her gaze wandered, fixed on a spot on the floor. Between sighs, she confessed to feeling like she was paying for sins, a weight she had carried from an early age as she witnessed her family face disagreements, drug use and financial difficulties. Eliza's anguish went beyond her own HIV status; it was a reflection on a vicious cycle of punishment that permeated her life and that of her loved ones. Eliza's narrative, permeated by a sense of fatality, brought back thoughts of the Buendía family from Gabriel García Márquez's "One Hundred Years of Solitude". The writer concludes the work with the intriguing phrase, "because the strains condemned to a hundred years of solitude didn't have a second chance on earth". This association made me think about how many people and families, unfortunately, can feel trapped in a cycle of adversity that seems destined to last. I found myself thinking that, beyond magical realism, how many families, in fact, are sadly doomed? What is my role in the face of a tragedy that seems to have been announced and expected by so many families? But I'll tell you later why I disagree with Gabriel García Márquez.

\*\*\*

In order to fulfill my role as a student and offer support to Eliza, I tried to better understand the dynamic between her and Ruan. Asking about their relationship, their aspirations, dreams and everyday aspects, Eliza revealed a close and affectionate bond with her son. She said that she is very close to Ruan and is actively involved in all aspects of his life. She said that Ruan has many friends, yet a shadow hangs over this apparent normality: none of his friends, and not all of his family, are aware of his HIV-positive status. Eliza's persistent fear is that disclosure will lead to some form of exclusion, even in contemporary times with wide access to information about HIV. In a moment of vulnerability, Eliza shared her deepest dream: she wants Ruan to achieve independence and follow his own path. However, even though she longs for him to walk life's journey alone, she confesses the difficulty in loosening this maternal bond. The sincere expression of her feelings reveals the complexity of motherhood in the face of adversity, suggesting a duality between the desire to allow her son autonomy and the fear of abandoning him after so many years of being an overprotective mother.

This revealing conversation highlights not only the practical challenges of Ruan's condition, but also the emotional struggles Eliza faces as a mother. In understanding the depth of these challenges, I realized the importance not only of the clinical aspect, but also of emotional support and building bridges to promote acceptance and inclusion, overcoming the stigma associated with HIV, often from the family itself.

But Ruan is not just a diagnosis: he is a boy immersed in the world of the arts. An active member of an artistic group, he has taken part in plays, attends drawing classes and has an affinity for dance and abstract drawings. Ruan is a young man from the world of ideas, as Plato would say. For Eliza, he represents not just a boy with a disease, but her most precious possession, coloring her world and giving a deep meaning to her existence. This portrait of Ruan highlights the richness of his personality and passions, making clear the importance of seeing the patient beyond medical conditions and valuing the uniqueness and potential of each individual.

I began to question her about emotional support over time, asking Eliza if she had ever considered seeking psychological assistance to deal with the complexity of her relationship and emotional dependence on Ruan. This turned out to be one of the most distressing moments of the conversation because, in my attempt to offer help, I noticed a possible momentary unease in Eliza. After I suggested therapy, she asked: "No, why? Do I need it?"

A question followed by a laugh shared between us. The lightness of Eliza's laughter dissipated some of the tension I felt at that moment. To soften the impact of the suggestion, I resorted to medical psychology concepts learned in my first year at university. I explained that it's not necessary for something to be wrong to seek the help of a psychologist. It can also be to maintain balance and preserve what is good. This preventative approach, focused on ongoing well-being, offered Eliza a new horizon. She expressed her willingness to see a psychologist as soon as possible, indicating an openness to considering the importance of mental health in her journey.

Another point I was instructed to ask about was the family support network, which is also very important for adherence and staying with long-term treatments such as HIV. With this in mind, I tried to understand Eliza and Ruan's relationship with his father and brother. When I asked her about her relationship with Ruan's father, Eliza was incisive: "I don't know and I don't want to know. It's just me and my son". This statement, although direct, showed Eliza's decision to preserve her own peace, erasing from her memory any trace of a past that could be painful. Her firm response conveyed the message that certain wounds did not need to be revisited, as they had already healed. During the conversation, Eliza shared an old photo, a relic from when her two children were babies. The image, now recently scribbled on by Ruan and his older brother, revealed an affectionate bond between the two. This expression of mutual affection was a source of pride for Eliza, noticeable even behind the masks that covered her smile. As she complimented them, highlighting the beauty of the babies in the photograph, Eliza leaned her head on her shoulder, proud of herself.

The feeling of having contributed to a moment of lightness and wonder in her journey was priceless. Eliza's proud gaze at the photograph reflected not only the love between her children, but also the resilience and strength that permeated her own journey as a mother. This episode highlighted the importance of recognizing and celebrating moments of joy and connection, even in the face of challenges. Amidst the masks that hid part of their expressions, the exchange of smiles and shared complicity reinforced the beauty present in simple moments of recognition and appreciation in Eliza's complex life. It really was an incredible feeling.

Here, I found myself reflecting on one of the greatest pillars of medicine, which appears in the Hippocratic Oath, which I will take in front of my family, teachers and colleagues when I finish my degree.

*"To heal when possible; to relieve when necessary; to console always."*

I feel that, even with a few years to go before I graduate, I have managed to put into practice this maxim that is at the heart of medical practice.

Towards the end of our conversation, Eliza shared one of the most difficult moments of her life: when Ruan, due to the virus, spent months with severe communication and locomotion difficulties. Even years after that episode, he still carries a sequel that limits the movement of one of his legs, which becomes a challenge for someone who loves to dance and communicate through his body. That's when Eliza, her eyes welling up with tears again, said that:

*"All I asked God for was to see him normal. If I had a study, I'd like to cure him".*

It was at that moment that I held back my tears as I thought of all the effort a mother makes to see her son well and to make his dreams come true. I remembered my own mother who, from a distance in another city, makes a huge effort to make me realize my dream of becoming a doctor one day. I thought that at that moment, it was up to me to play the role of the person who recognizes all the work and concern that Eliza has had for her son.

With empathy, I explained to Eliza about the accessible and quality treatments offered by the Brazilian health system, pointing out that both of them, with undetectable viral loads, enjoy a practically normal life in control of the virus. Asking permission, I held her hand, fixed my gaze on hers and shared that I can only imagine how challenging it must be to live her reality. I reinforced the message that she is not alone, emphasizing that her and Ruan's follow-up is a joint effort between patient and doctors. I emphasized that neither she nor the health professionals are solely responsible, but rather partners in this process, cultivating a doctor-patient relationship based on transparency and collaboration. This approach sought to provide comfort and reinforce the importance of mutual support in Eliza and Ruan's journey.

After this moment of intense emotion with Eliza, I felt the need to take a short break for both of us, to get her a glass of water. As I walked down the corridor towards the water fountain, I saw my colleague engaged in a conversation with one of the children who would probably be seen soon. He looked at me like he was in a moment of mutual learning, a deep connection between student and patient. When I returned to the room with the glass of water, I realized that Eliza was already a little more emotionally stable. However, she chose to leave the glass on the table without touching it, perhaps reluctant to remove the mask to drink. This simple, seemingly insignificant gesture reflected the complexity of the emotions and situation we were facing. The constant presence of the masks during the conversation, as well as being a precautionary measure in the midst of the pandemic, became a symbol of the barrier between us and the vulnerability shared by Eliza. The glass of water, offered as a gesture of care, remained untouched, highlighting the delicacy needed when dealing with the emotions exposed during our conversation.

This brief episode in the corridor, marked by the shared glances between my colleague with the child and me, reinforced the idea that, even in busy clinical environments, there is room to learn from every interaction. Each patient, whether a mother like Eliza or a child waiting for care, has valuable lessons to offer, challenging us to cultivate a deeper understanding of the human experience. The experience reinforced the importance not only of addressing patients' medical needs, but also of recognizing the emotional and social complexities that permeate the clinical environment. The symbolic gesture of the glass of water, even though it wasn't consumed, represented an attempt to nourish not only the body, but also the soul.

\*\*\*

The experience with Eliza not only enriched the more human dimension of my student-patient relationship, but also allowed me to deeply re-evaluate concepts previously ingrained in me. In particular, it questioned a notion that I perceive still haunts many junior doctors, myself included, when they enter medical school: the ego. This quest for absolute control and aversion to death, especially when facing non-curable situations, are aspects that I have noticed shape the medical imagination. The experience with Eliza served as a catalyst for rethinking and challenging these conceptions, offering a more compassionate and realistic perspective on the complexity inherent in medical practice.

I notice that, in addition to preferences for more clinical or surgical approaches, the choice of a medical specialty to follow is often permeated by the desire to achieve curative results. There is an inclination to consider that only the complete cure of a disease is a satisfactory and worthy outcome. Although the desire to fix and solve problems is a characteristic shared by those who choose medicine, I realize that the perspective in relation to this can directly impact the doctor-patient dynamic.

It is crucial to recognize that medicine covers a wide range of challenges and situations, often going beyond the ability to provide a definitive cure. Developing a more holistic understanding, valuing effective management, quality of life and emotional support, can enrich medical practice. This perspective not only reflects the complexity of clinical reality, but also strengthens the connection and understanding between doctor and patient, especially in cases where a complete cure may not be a viable possibility.

As I've said before, I believe that the doctor's primary function, in line with the principles of Hippocrates, is, above all, to improve the patient's quality of life, not just to seek a cure. I recognize that dealing with the feeling of powerlessness in the face of a disease that is still incurable or an irreversible process is challenging. However, I see this situation as a unique opportunity for students and doctors to talk to their own ego. It is essential that we understand that, although we are often charged by society to act as omnipotent, medicine is not an exact science and we cannot always offer definitive solutions. Facing this aspect of medical practice not only demands humility, but also opens up space to explore other dimensions of care, regardless of whether a complete cure is a possibility. This approach reinforces the essence of medicine as a profession centered on caring for the person and humanization, transcending the mere search for curative results.

After experiencing the neurology rotation in the fourth year of college, combined with experiences with patients like Eliza, facing diseases that were not curable but were susceptible to dignified longitudinal therapies, I decided to pursue the specialty of neurology. This journey has reinforced my commitment to providing continuous support and compassionate care, recognizing that even in the face of therapeutic limitations, it is possible to contribute to a meaningful and quality life for those facing neurological challenges.

Having taken part in various conversations with patients with HIV, Multiple Sclerosis and other diseases that, as yet, have no cure, has made me realize that a person or their family is not destined for a solitary existence, reflecting the sad fate of the Buendías in Gabriel García Márquez's novel. I understand that our role as health professionals goes beyond the search for a cure; it is, above all, to offer warmth and comfort so that our patients can live as well as possible, considering their circumstances. I recognize the limitations of medicine in the face of certain conditions, such as in the case of neurological patients, where a definitive cure can be an unattainable goal. However, this awareness does not diminish my satisfaction in providing hope and contributing to the quality of life of these individuals. Knowing that I won't be able to cure all neurological cases doesn't discourage me, as my focus is on the possibility of witnessing meaningful moments in their lives.

I believe that every hug, every piece of abstract art and every scribble on a photo are valuable expressions of affection and vitality. They are gestures that transcend physical limitations and reinforce the humanity of each patient. Maintaining this perspective is fundamental to preserving dignity and hope, not just during medical appointments, but throughout the course of these people's lives. Our mission, then, is to provide support, understanding and an environment that allows patients to embrace life with meaning, even in the face of adversity.

When I chose medicine, my central desire was to cultivate a deep doctor-patient relationship. However, when I started the course, I was confronted with the scarcity of opportunities to improve or even minimally practice this aspect. As we progressed through the course, this finding was corroborated, echoing the findings of the well-known study "The Devil is in the Third Year: A Longitudinal Study of Erosion of Empathy in Medical Study". The academic path often leads us to a gradual loss of empathy, prioritizing quick, objective care over a deeper connection with the patient. This contrast between the initial aspiration and the reality of the course led me to reflect on how we can reintegrate empathy more meaningfully into medical teaching and practice.

I believe that it is vitally important for the training of every doctor and health professional to have opportunities, throughout their academic journey, to conduct more subjective anamneses, centered on the patient and not just on the disease. The practice of writing about subjective experiences should be commonplace in medical courses, since the profession is, above all, centered on human relationships. This more global approach allows students to deepen their understanding of the patient as a unique being, involving not only physical symptoms, but also emotional, social and cultural aspects that impact on their health. Cultivating this skill from the early years of training not only nurtures empathy and understanding, but also contributes to building more complete professionals, capable of offering more comprehensive and humane care to patients.

As for human relations in medicine, I believe that developing soft skills is the most valuable skill to exercise and polish. This competence encompasses empathy, effective communication and an understanding of patients' emotional needs, essential elements for shaping a medical practice centered on human care. In contrast, even with significant advances in artificial intelligence, there are intrinsic aspects of the doctor-patient relationship that cannot be authentically replicated by machines.

The complexity of human emotions, the nuances of interpersonal interactions and the ability to interpret not only physical symptoms, but also emotional and social contexts, are elements that defy complete replacement by artificial intelligence. Empathy, in particular, is a profoundly human quality, based on experiences, understanding and emotional connections that transcend the capacity of machines. The trust, comfort and security that a patient gains from interacting with a human doctor are products of genuine communication and holistic understanding, crucial elements that highlight the irreplaceability of the human touch in medical practice.

After our conversation, Ruan expressed his desire to continue dancing and began a professional journey creating graphic designs on the computer. Eliza, for her part, decided to take up the hobby of practicing street dance. The end of the conversation was marked by a warm hug from Eliza, who expressed her gratitude for the opportunity to share thoughts she had never revealed before, not even to herself. From that day on, I realized that I had made the right choice for my life. Watching Ruan and Eliza's horizons change, unfolding into new aspirations and activities, reinforced the importance of medical care that transcends the limits of physiology. For me, medicine is not just about diagnosing and treating illnesses, but about promoting quality of life and the emotional well-being of patients.

The positive impact on Ruan and Eliza's choices highlighted how narrative medicine can be a powerful tool for reconnecting patients with themselves and their passions, contributing to a more holistic approach to health. Eliza's heartfelt hug and expression of gratitude were a vivid testimony to the importance of listening to, understanding and sharing patients' stories. This experience solidified my conviction that choosing narrative medicine as an integral part of my medical journey was indeed the right choice. By providing a space for personal narratives to emerge, we can positively influence not only patients' physical condition, but also their emotional journey and the way they perceive life itself.

Finally, I'm curious to know which roles Ruan most enjoyed playing, or which artists were his favorites. I hope the next hundred years of his and his mother's lives are filled with all good things, except solitude.

# As Much an Art as It Is a Science

Dikshya Parajuli
University of Otago Medical School
New Zealand

*"Inferior STEMI, 87 y/o female. Metastatic cancer, recent aortic dissection. Do not resuscitate, for palliative cares only"* cubicle three's ambulance notes read.

I was on my emergency medicine placement as a final year medical student. I strolled over to cubicle three, where an elderly female who I'll refer to as Edna met my gaze with glassy eyes and a tired smile. Her emaciated body was surrounded by doctors and several nurses. She had been discharged from hospital back to her rest home for end of life cares only three days prior. With widespread breast cancer metastases, she was on huge doses of opioids and had been under the care of hospice for some time. After an episode of unrelenting chest pain that morning, Edna had decided it was all too much and had asked to return to hospital for what would inevitably be her final days.

When questioned by the doctor as to why she wanted to die in hospital and not her own space, Edna replied *"I feel more safe dying here. I will get better care here"*. She spoke with poise and certainty. Tinged with the acceptance of a life well lived, she possessed no denial in the futility of further medical treatment. Although her organs were failing, her desire to maintain dignity over the body that remained was still burning fiercely. She wanted to die with dignity. In a place she felt safe. *Safe to die.*

A nurse walked in with a vital signs monitor, and immediately turned around on hearing the doctor say *"no observations, she's palliative"*. The doctor's words and the nurse's actions appeared so devoid of emotion. One by one, everyone left. A room that seconds prior had been full of minds skilled and dedicated to *save lives* was abruptly empty, leaving only a dying patient and a medical student behind.

Edna's enfeebled skeleton was visibly exhausted. As she lay there in tremendous discomfort, the weight of her suffering became palpable. The knowledge I was armed with on the clinical aspects of her presentation felt not only inapplicable, but brutally irrelevant to the visceral nature of her suffering. Medical school had taught me about many ways to keep a patient alive, but very little about how to comfort them as they die. I felt idealistic, inexperienced and unprepared for the strength of my own emotions.

Edna's desire for someone's emotional presence was obvious. As her youth filled eyes turned to me, uncertainty engulfed my mind. For a moment, I wondered if I even belonged in the room. A familiar feeling of unease took hold, as if I was suddenly swimming in waters out of my depth. I had spent the last several years learning the intricacies of human biology, disease and pathology. I had worked hard to develop my clinical competence and confidence. I had a lot of theoretical knowledge. However, when face-to-face with a dying soul for whose illness an obvious panacea did not exist, I felt *helpless*. I longed to swim back to shallower water.

*"Not a very exciting one is it?"* one of the ED doctors asked me as I walked over to prepare a cup of tea. Determined to not let him see the tears that I was fighting back, I nodded and with tea in my hands, I walked back to Edna's room. Though I felt like there was little I could do for Edna, the thought of leaving her alone in that cubicle ached me. My presence emerged as the only solace I could offer her. I handed her the warm drink and accompanied her as I waited for her palliative care team to take over care. Maybe I was merely treading water, but I felt driven by a naïve urge to extend empathy and a desire to diminish discomfort.

Whilst we waited, Edna drank her tea and shared with me her wishes and worries. In that time, I saw Edna's fear turn into trust – trust that although her illness could not be reversed and her life could not be saved, she *could* and *would* be cared for here. An unspoken bond had formed between us, instilling a sense of trust and vulnerability that transcended the limitations of clinical interventions. I realised then that even as a medical student, I was and could continue becoming someone who belonged in the room.

Eventually, an orderly from the patient transfer services came to transfer Edna to the west wing of the medical ward. The place where comfort cares would be initiated for her. A place where death would neither be hastened *nor* postponed, where she would get the dignified ending she so deeply desired.

Over the next few days, I continued to visit Edna. I soon learnt that apart from her palliative care team, I was her only regular visitor.

Each time I entered her room, her glistening eyes would turn to me, beseeching me as to whether I had any time to lend her. Any length of undivided empathetic presence was enough to make her smile. On days I had time, I would sit down to her level, and I would listen. On days I didn't, I would pop in, say hello, top up her water, open her window; do *anything* to remind her that she had not been forgotten.

And each time I left, I would close the curtains that separated her from the chaos of the medical ward. Though flimsy and fragile, the curtains preserved Edna's dignity. *Dignity is all she wanted,* I would remind myself.

Just as the flowers on her windowsill that slowly began to wilt, Edna grew weaker and weaker with each passing day; her wrinkles becoming more defined, her breathing becoming more laboured. Her medical progress notes validated my observations that every organ in her body was slowly withdrawing *bit by bit* from life. Watching Edna dwindle amidst a backdrop of withering flowers served as a sobering reminder that death is an inevitable part of every life cycle. Someday, we all approach an end. No matter how resisted and refused, death is the most certain thing in *all* of life.

Each sunset does *not* bring the promise of a new dawn.
Everything, including life itself, is temporary.

Over the days I visited Edna, mortality became less of an abstract concept and more of a defined and truthful reality.

Some consultants treat ward rounds like an authoritative and ritualistic task; towering over patients, reciting questions on autopilot and hurriedly running off to their next review. The patient meek or mute, trusting the doctor wholeheartedly, ready to bear whatever suffering was necessary.

Edna's palliative care doctor on the other hand, was the opposite. By weaving together strands of empathy, expertise and experience, she treated her time with Edna not as a compulsory task, but rather an opportunity to forge a relationship founded on understanding. She listened and acknowledged, and by doing so she made Edna feel seen and heard. She found out what was important to Edna and fought hard to respect her wishes. It was as if she deeply understood that although she would not save Edna's life, by virtue of her actions alone, she *could* become a conduit for healing. She was simply incredible.

As I watched her truly care for Edna, I could not help but reflect on how throughout my entire academic career, I had been trained to value objective performance. Grades, numbers and percentages had equated to progress and the promise that I could be a good doctor. However, in the face of Edna's insurmountable suffering, the skill that appeared to matter the most was the very one that had never been assessed or taught objectively; *empathy*. At this realisation, medical school felt like a dress rehearsal for the real responsibility that lay ahead in my future as a doctor.

On one of my morning visits, Edna whispered *"Can you spare me a little longer today, dear?"*.

My emotions, which had already begun retreating inwards at noticing how much weaker she looked, were acutely wrenched back into the present. Her desire for someone's emotional presence was tangible. I looked down at my clipboard; a long list of uncompleted academic tasks glanced back at me. However, the only thing that felt right in that moment was to sit by Edna's side. As a student, I had something that her doctors did not. *I had time.* And there **were** things I could learn, even from a dying patient.

I smiled, sat down and turned away my clipboard.

That day, Edna recounted a vibrant timeline of her life's events. From college, to family, love, parenthood, illness and age, I learnt many things about the magnificent tapestry that had been her life; the rich and royal hue with which her 87 years had been woven. The lucidity of her recollections served as a poignant reminder that patients at the end of life *are still living*. Whilst a component of their individuality becomes lost the minute we exchange their clothes for a hospital gown, and their name for a room number; they are still individuals with stories, identities *and* emotions.

As I listened to Edna, I found myself questioning who I was to witness her at this moment, *the most fragile and vulnerable she had been in all of her life*. I recalled a quote from Dr Paul Kalanithi's book *When Breath Becomes Air; "All of medicine, not just cadaver dissections, trespasses into sacred spheres"*. In that moment, I felt like I had finally grasped the essence of Dr Kalanithi's message. Perhaps this is what was meant to be taught in the *hidden curriculum* mentioned repeatedly in medical school.

I genuinely think Edna realised how truly privileged I felt to be in her presence and to give her the gift of my time, and I think she also understood that she was giving me a lot too. It was as if she already knew that although this was the end of her, it was only the beginning for me. The beginning of a career in service and I think she could see that I was determined to learn how to serve well.

I visited Edna again the day before my two week vacation. A sense of vacuity settled into my stomach as I realised then that it was my time to say goodbye – *goodbye, forever*. Despite knowing all too well that it would likely be the last time I would ever see her, I could not bring myself to tell her this.

A kaleidoscope of emotions crept in and took root within – sadness, guilt, fear and frustration. Unsure of how to navigate the balance between being professional and being human, I loitered next to Edna like a shadow. Visible, but not fully present. Paralysed by the thought that I might say or do something wrong. Never before had I farewelled a dying patient. Abruptly, I was in uncharted waters, in unfamiliar territory. However, this was a first like no other. I found myself wondering if there was room for humanism and empathy in this stoic profession that by default fosters distance and emotional detachment. As my mind searched for answers, I felt tears well up in my eyes, and slowly drift into my respirator mask. A subtle expression of connection that inherently felt bold, an expression of what it means to be human. Unable to hold Edna's gaze, I turned to face the window, her withering flowers framing the periphery of my blurry vision.
I said goodbye like any other day, daring hard to not lull my words with a sense of finality. I remember wishing that day that I could have been half as strong-willed and composed as Edna had appeared.

I never saw Edna again.

On my first day back after my vacation, I made my way up to the west wing of the medical ward where I had walked many times to visit Edna. I probably could have walked that route in my sleep. However, this time, the room label outside Edna's room had a new name on it. My shock initially became confusion, and then turned into discomfort. Her absence became acutely apparent.

A nurse who had regularly cared for Edna walked past and confirmed for me what I already knew deep down. I learnt from her that Edna had died two days ago. She told me that Edna had been comfortable at the time of her passing and right throughout, she had received care that aligned with her values, guided by a doctor whose only goal was to respect these. All of her wishes had been honoured. *"It was the dignified death that Edna had wanted all along"* The nurse said softly.

Upon hearing this, the pangs of sadness and guilt I felt slowly lifted and I found myself smiling.

In medical school, we have been reminded time and time again by our professors, tutors and lecturers that our best teachers will *always* be our patients. I have never once doubted this, for knowledge delivered to me about suffering and illness has paled in comparison to the lessons I have gained from directly witnessing, comforting and caring for patients. Edna reaffirmed this understanding in every aspect.

My encounter with Edna was deeply moving and served as a raw illustration of nuances of the human condition; life, emotion, identity and death. Confronted with the fragility of life and bearing witness to the suffering of a dying woman whose fate that could not be changed, I found myself searching deeply for ways to alleviate her suffering but realised that time and empathy were the only things I could offer. The profound connection I built with Edna has forever coloured how I view the purpose of my profession; medicine is more than just the privilege of saving lives, it is also the privilege of attenuating pain and suffering even when lives cannot be saved.

Witnessing the joy my visits brought Edna shattered an illusion I had naïvely and unconsciously crafted as a medical student; that caring for patients meant solely *fixing* problems. After all, as doctors we are trained to fix and solve. Our identities are formed on our ability to cure. The corollary, therefore, is that a failure to *cure*, is a failure to *care*. However, Edna taught me that patients are not merely broken objects that require fixing and death is not always a failure. Nor is death always a battle, at least not one that we can always win.

Through the act of holding space for empathy and compassion for Edna, I realised how transformative these values can be when helping patients navigate the difficult terrain of emotions presented by illness. When I had first met Edna in the emergency room, the interactions between her and healthcare providers in the department had appeared to lack emotion. In a field where exposure to pain and suffering forms the crux of virtually every encounter, it is not surprising that healthcare professionals sometimes subconsciously engage in a degree of emotional desensitisation. Perhaps a means of self-protection, detachment helps us to not feel too deeply for patients who are hurting, and especially those who *cannot* be healed.

However, complete emotional disengagement, particularly when interacting with those at the end of life, diminishes our ability to care and is contrary to our promise to *do no harm*. In such a sacred space, expressing anything other than compassion *feels* inhumane. And this *is* okay – as long as we have processes by which to let go of this emotional residue and mitigate compassion exhaustion.

We owe empathy to those whose health is entrusted to us. Whilst they live, whilst they suffer *and* whilst they die.

The physician-patient relationship is a unique one and interactions between the two tread on a delicate tightrope – an intricate juxtaposition of science *and* art, of opportunity *and* obligation, of professionalism *and* humanity. I am constantly awed by the vulnerability and trust patients endow upon physicians. In palliative medicine, the connection we get to form with patients feels even more raw; in this space, connection has the potential to alleviate suffering in ways that pills and ventilators *cannot*.

In the realm of end of life care, both fortes and deficiencies of clinicians become exaggerated. Throughout my clinical years, I have seen many times where a patient's death has brought clinicians a deep and palpable sense of defeat, despite their death being expected *and* inevitable. The heaviest burden of the clinician's deficiency in these cases fell on those whose lives and identities were already under threat; for it was the patient who was subjected to further suffering and undignified interventions for minimal gain in their quality or quantity of life. A diminished ability to accept death and dying as meaningful aspects of life sometimes drive clinicians to cure-driven interventions and futile prolongation of life. Though modern medicine is captivating, powerful and has tremendous capacity to heal, at times it also strives for life *at all costs*.

I cannot help but wonder what difference might have been made to those patients' lives if their clinician's had recognised that their role was not to *fight* fate, but simply to improve the quality of their patients' lives, for as long as their lives existed. In those moments, I remember wishing desperately that they could have had a death like Edna's.

On the contrary, I have also had the privilege of witnessing doctors deliver timely, high-quality and holistic care to palliative patients; care that was directly concordant with patient values *and* priorities. These physicians treated their patients as people, and not merely problems to be solved. They cared for their patients deeply, even when giving them life-altering diagnoses. They stood by their patients' side as they came to make sense of their illness, reshaped their identities and made difficult decisions about what kind of life was worth living. They were empathetic, eloquent and passionate to do right by those they were caring for. Edna's palliative care doctor did all of these things.

These doctors showed me that engaging in our own humanity in service of our patients is not only possible *but necessary*.
They fuelled my desire to learn not only how to *fix,* but also how to *care.* They taught me that compassion does not need to be dispensed frugally out of fear of blurring the boundaries of the physician-patient relationship and that being good at this work does not require the suppression of our humanity, but rather the expansion of it.

During my time in paediatrics, I had a few days of placement in the regional neonatal intensive care unit (NICU). End of life discussions took on a different moral lens when they were not about 87 year old individuals who were rendered a life-limiting diagnosis, but rather cherished premature infants who were at the *beginning* of life. The neonatologists at the unit however delivered exemplary care; they guided families through difficult shared decision-making and they navigated the ethical dilemmas of futile care with equipoise and moral clarity. I was simply in awe of them. *How did they know which lives could be saved, which lives couldn't and which lives shouldn't? Like me, did they too take home the suffering and sadness exuded by families who had lost a loved one too soon?* Surrounded by tens of infant incubators, each attempting to provide a budding life with a second womb, I would often find myself questioning whether I would ever learn to lead and live with such responsibility, or if I was even cut out for the tremendous responsibility of medicine. My time in the NICU left me pondering many questions, but it left me certain of one fact; that doing this profession the justice it deserves would require more than only clinical excellence. If medicine truly is a moral endeavour and its goal is to truly care for people – then I needed to develop more than just my knowledge. As such, learning how to balance the science and art of this sacred profession has become not merely an aspiration for me, but an imperative.

Every time I reflect on what I have learnt from these incredible clinicians, I feel a deep sense of respect and appreciation for my future colleagues in medicine and a newfound motivation to grow into a doctor who one day can care for patients exactly as I have seen them do.

Palliative medicine has led me to the end of many lives and in doing so has uniquely highlighted the power of informed choice. Some patients will consent to any intervention or drug, if it gives them any chance of a longer life. Others think instantly about what kind of life is worth living for them, and will forgo quantity for quality. As clinicians, we may have the knowledge and expertise to manage illnesses, but it is not up to us to single-handedly make decisions about what level of care is enough. We may not always be able to save our patients lives, but we can and should ask questions to understand our patients wishes, values and priorities for care. Nathan reminded me of this.

Nathan was a 25 year old male I met on the same emergency rotation I had met Edna. He had a rare form of epithelioid sarcoma with pleural metastases and bilateral pneumothoraces. At a very early stage in his cancer journey, Nathan had been offered surgery and radiation therapy – both of which he had declined due to religious beliefs. His past admission notes were complex – with strands of ethics, illness and self-determination interwoven to create tension between the principles of beneficence and autonomy. However, it was deemed that Nathan had full decision-making capacity and that he understood the consequences of his choices. As such, his ultimate right to refuse treatment was respected. Now, the ceiling of treatment for Nathan was palliative – health professionals caring for him would do everything to keep him comfortable, but would not actively treat his illness or aggressively manage him if he was to become more unwell. And this was exactly the kind of care that aligned with Nathan's wishes, values and beliefs. This is all Nathan wanted.

I once heard him listlessly explain to a healthcare assistant who had questioned his choices whilst nursing his wounds, *"My life is not truly mine without me, and with this cancer, I am not me"*.

When I first was introduced to Nathan's story, I was initially taken aback by how someone so young had chosen to forgo beneficial treatment and allow cancer to invade his body. In the context of young Nathan's inevitable death, I could not help but think about the vastness of the chasm between the life he may have had if he had consented to cancer treatment, and the life he would soon no longer have because of his choices. The vastness of this chasm served as a powerful reminder to me that whilst patients have the right to life, they also have the right to be autonomous and make decisions about what kind of care they wish to receive. Healthcare providers have a duty to do everything they can to provide beneficent care and to first, *do no harm*, but competent, fully informed patients, ***can*** refuse standard medical care. Nathan reminded me that there is more to living than just being *alive*.

As doctors we are the doers, the ones who act; as patients, we are simply done and acted upon. When we are the ones who act, we may have an idea of what it is like to be a patient, but most of the time, we do not know what it is *really* like. I personally came to first grapple with this realisation only a few months ago when I too traversed the line from being on the side where one acts, to being on the side where one is acted *upon*.

Earlier this year, my ten year old younger sister was abruptly ill with an acute abdomen and required two emergency surgeries back to back in the span of a few days. At the time, I was miles from home and in the midst of a busy medical rotation. However, on hearing the news, I requested urgent leave and caught the next flight home. Little did I realise at the time that this would be one of the most difficult times in my life as a sibling, and one of the most *transformative* as a student doctor.

Throughout my years at medical school, I had made trips to the operating room and watched the induction of general anaesthesia at least a hundred times. I could recite the intricate details of the stages of *induction, maintenance* and *emergence.* However, when I walked my sister in for her emergency laparotomy, I was now on the other side of the operating table, the other side of the anaesthetist's needle and the consent documents. In that space, every word and every action of the medical practitioners surrounding me seemed to carry with it a different mountain of significance. The power imbalance between the patient, and the doctor has never been so evident.

*How little do we understand the ordeals we subject our patients to?* I found myself wondering. I recalled learning in third year medical humanities that the English word *patient* originally stemmed from the Latin term *patiens,* meaning '*the one who suffers and endures'.* The present particle of the verb, *patior,* translated into *'I am suffering'.* This time, it was my sister and I who were suffering, and it felt visceral. I ached to my core.

As a student in the operating room, I was very calm and level-headed. As a family member of a patient, I was fearful and weak. As I watched the sedative drugs take effect over my sister, my heart trembled with each beat. My eyes could no longer see clear through the dusk of tears that flowed unrestrained. The last thing my sister asked me before succumbing to the unopposed effect of propofol was *"Sis, will the surgery hurt?"*.

I was then ushered out of the operating room. The two hours whilst I waited for her to come out of her operation felt like a lifetime. In those moments, the remainder of the world ceased to exist in my fragile recollection. My vast existential worries, deadlines and tasks became infinitesimal. Time passed slowly as I waited for her to come out of her operation.

I spent the next three weeks by her bedside, attending to her every need. Feeding her, braiding her hair, helping her as she relearned how to walk and play again. As a medical student, I was trained to view suffering through a professional lens; I was trained to cure. However, when faced with a loved one's illness, I naturally assumed my role of a caregiver; entwined with heartfelt emotions – fear, hope, love and deep yearning for recovery.

Thankfully my sister was okay. She continued to make triumphs in her recovery in every aspect and after 24 days in hospital, she was on her way back home; her laparotomy and laparoscopy surgical sites appearing insignificant in the grand scheme of the suffering she had endured. She is now healthy, happy and is healing at home and I feel blessed beyond belief to have her with me. What I learnt from my experience as a family member watching a loved one navigate the challenges of illness will always be an unshakable part of my foundation, informing a myriad of future learning and a relentless drive to serve others with compassion as a medical practitioner.

Although I was constantly surrounded by stories of suffering in my academic life, it was when suffering infiltrated into my personal life that the tenuousness and fragility of life became profoundly obvious. In that brutally painful period of my life, I too drowned in the labyrinth of emotions I had seen patients and their families navigate amidst illness many times before. It was in that space that I came to understand through direct experience that firstly, that privilege and responsibility go hand in hand and secondly, illness evokes some of the darkest days a patient and their families will ever see.

Illness and death are certain in life for no one is exempt from humanity's ultimate destination. However as doctors, we have the opportunity of honouring and respecting these processes, and transforming something that is unavoidably painful and devastating into a meaningful life event. We may even be able to plant seeds of empowerment. In this space, we hold immense power to alleviate fear, suffering and pain that patients and their families experience. What an immense privilege this is.

Processing my encounter with Edna has given me the opportunity to reflect on many thought-provoking patient interactions I have encountered as a medical student. Undoubtedly, witnessing patients at their most weakest and vulnerable comes with emotional costs. There were days where I do not know where to even begin unpacking the complex emotions born out from my time on placement. There were times where I too took home the turmoil I see patients and their families face. There were moments of uncertainty, fear and confusion I found myself reliving.

However, through such experiences, I have discovered a shared vulnerability that unifies me to patients I have learned from and cared for; whose beautiful, sometimes painful narratives I have had the privilege of immersing myself into. Such challenges have also offered me the opportunity to cultivate a repertoire of strategies to cope with the challenges of this work, which I will no doubt use in my future as a junior doctor. I have learnt to ask for advice from my seniors when in need, to take time to debrief, cherish my time with loved ones and to look after my own wellbeing. In doing so, I am learning how to care for myself better, whilst I learn how to care for others.

Through the mundanity and intensity of it all, I have not once questioned why I chose this career or whether it would be worth it. Medicine, rich with its complex emotions and responsibilities, is *absolutely* what I want to do. Encounters with patients like Edna humbly remind me of this.

Even months later, I still find myself wondering about Edna. On the day she arrived into the emergency room, she knew that she likely had days to maybe weeks to live. She was constantly aware of her mortality, but she did not seem to fear it once. She taught me a little about dying, but a lot more about living.

Months later and I continue to feel immense gratitude for all that she taught me during her final days. Because of Edna, I have in fact truly come to appreciate patients, their experiences of illness and stories of suffering as both windows *and* mirrors. Windows to better understand intrinsic aspects of the human condition; biology, mortality and suffering, mirrors to provide a platform for deep moral reflection and a glimpse of the moral dimension of our sacred profession. Patients give us the unique privilege of both *seeing out* and *seeing in;* they offer new understandings, whilst offering reflections.

I will always remember Edna. I'll remember how her aged skin starkly contrasted her eternal youth-filled eyes. I'll remember how she shared the most special parts of her humble life story with me; for me to learn from and to cherish. I'll remember her vulnerability, her integrity and above all; her desire for dignity.

Thank you Edna for being both a window *and* a mirror. You deepened my understanding of the science and art of medicine, and you also gave deeper meaning to my own sense of place within it.
I see you in every 87 year old I have seen since, in every dying patient who does not have family at their bedside and in every palliative individual who faces death with strength. It has been months since I first met you, but I have still not stopped learning from you.

Because of you, I now find myself taking more time with my patients, seeking to understand the experience of their illness, not just their symptoms.
I aim to listen, without rushing.
I allow my patients to teach me to *see out* and *see in.*
I err increasingly, on the side of *compassion.*
I try really hard to not become too emotionally detached that I lose touch with humanity, and not too emotionally involved that I lose my ability to assess objectively.
I embrace the notion that caring extends beyond curing.
I slow down and make time for patients so they too, like you, feel seen and heard.

These actions, though small, are helping me to build a humanistic perspective into my craft of doctoring. As I progress further on in my medical journey and closer to becoming a doctor, actions that seek to achieve humanisation feel equally as important as clinical aptitude.

In learning that this work is sacred, and is as much art as it is science, I feel humbled and honoured by the opportunity to pursue a career in caring and aspire to do right by those whose health is placed upon my hands.

Caring for patients, particularly in the face of overwhelming suffering and at the end of life can be painful and raw, and it is a *huge* privilege. Thank you Edna, sincerely, for letting me be a part of your ending, and for shining a new light to the power of empathy and the art that is medicine.

# Chapter 1

# 1.1   The Ethics of Balint Work: Making the Kinship of Humanity Evident

Edith Katherine Knowlton, PhD
University of Washington
Department of Family Medicine
Seattle, Washington, USA
tryekk@aol.com

## Abstract

Though we do not use religion to differentiate the members of a Balint group, like other aspects of identity it is likely to be present and unnamed, making it a source of unspoken assumptions or attitudes which may affect a treatment relationship. Within the group religious differences may be contentious or powerful at closing down open minds. However, Balint groups are a great example of the well-researched finding that diversity enhances creativity and learning. This enhancing effect is as likely to be true for diversity of religion as for other identifiers. While our group focus and norms help to transcend differences which could be divisive, the very structure of Balint groups may help them bridge religious differences through parallels between the group work and the golden rule.   Current scholarship on ethics underscores the golden rule's lifelong applicability to situations of growing sophistication, from the playground to the operating room. Moreover, its near-universality among wisdom traditions and its ability to catalyze moral development make it a strong support of inclusiveness.  This paper considers different levels of development expressed in Balint groups; the group's ability to work with varying levels; and the processes involved in a Balint group's prompting of moral development.

When the American Balint Society surveyed its members in 2016, we found that our strongest diversity was in the area of religion or spirituality. We offered people six possible religions to claim. And we allowed folks to spell out their own alternative. So many people described themselves uniquely that we ended up with 26 categories. We did not consider this diversity as a challenge to the cohesion of the Society. On the contrary, we accepted the paradox that varied viewpoints can result in a more effective and coherent group (Chamorro-Premuzic, 2017).

Sternlieb (2018) looked at aspects of Balint culture that support diversity. The leaders' "encouragement of diverse contributions, valuing a range of emotional reactions, and an acceptance and integration of all contributions" create an atmosphere in which "[a]ll responses can inform the group about the case." And that atmosphere may soften the competitiveness and judgment professionals are likely to have overlearned, since "the focus on emotional responses creates a level or horizontal field of equal contributions among group members rather than the verticality of judgment attributed to smart responses or by virtue of one's position in a hierarchy."

By welcoming the differences in professional roles, personal styles, and the selves we bring to the group we are able to enrich Balint work. I suspect one ingredient of the secret sauce that makes Intensives so wonderful is the fact that those groups are as heterogeneous as we can make them. We do ask registrants about their professional roles and experience in Balint groups to help with that determination of heterogeneity. We do not ask about gender identification, country of origin, ethnicity or religion, the things our majority culture tends to use to sort people into categories of the deserving and undeserving, because we want to be clear we do not do that kind of sorting ourselves.

Religion has no official place in Balint groups, yet even without yarmulkas, crosses, headscarves or other indicia to signal varied affiliation, it sometimes comes up, and as we learned in our survey, it may be something Balint group members care deeply about. The presenter may say, "I grew up in a home with [my patient's] kind of religion." Or "I keep expecting to see my patient in my congregation." Like the other sources of variety religion is always there, whether talked about or not, as are our assumptions about religions. Those assumptions are unlikely to be wholly benign. As one person told me, "I was raised to be respectful of all faiths, but we understood ours was the real thing; the others were kind of fake fur."

This paper explores a parallel between Balint work and ethical thinking that transcends religious differences and whittles them down to size in important ways. It is not necessary for anyone in a group to be explicitly affiliated with a religion in order for the work to speak to whatever wisdom traditions happen to be represented. The areligious may be wedded to their views as well, so it is important that whatever the spiritual identifications of those present, the Balint group will speak to them.

This robust spiritual relevance can be understood by appreciating how the structure of the Balint group parallels the structure of the golden rule. If you are surprised by the rule's relevance to the complex contexts we discuss, please suspend your judgment for a bit. As philosopher Jeffrey Wattles (1996) concluded in his book on the subject, "The more deeply the golden rule is grasped, the less it seems a simple answer." (p. 189)

The basic questions of a Balint group are: What is it like to be this patient? What is the patient's experience? What is it like to be the practitioner for this person? What is the practitioner's experience? What is going on in their relationship?

The basic structure of the Golden Rule can also be read as calling for three actions. For example, the formulation "Love your neighbor as yourself" calls for 1.) loving one's neighbor; 2.) loving oneself; 3.) making the two equivalent or reciprocal. The formulation "do unto others as you would have others do unto you," works just as well:

The rule begins by setting forth the way the self wants to be treated as a standard of conduct; but by placing the other on a par with the self, the rule engages one in approximating a higher perspective from which the kinship of humanity is evident. (Wattles, 1996, p. 189)

Each of the actions required by the golden rule may be difficult and may call for extra effort. The Balint group provides a place for that effort and many minds to make that effort together. If I have disappointed myself in a professional encounter, the group may help me see my shortcoming more clearly or usefully. If my patient is baffling or makes me despair, the group may make him more interesting, more understandable or easier to care for anyway. And maybe there will be a point when my rightness fades to insignificance beside our common vulnerability or my need to serve does not require my patient to be servable as we muddle through.

Two aspects of the golden rule add to its power: first, it appears in some form in a myriad of religions and wisdom traditions. It has foundational relevance in indigenous, Judeo-Christian, and Asian traditions. The most encompassing exposition I could find offers eighteen different sources, including all widely ascribed faiths, First Nations, Wicca, and humanism. This makes the golden rule an excellent center pole for a most inclusive tent.

The other powerful aspect of the golden rule is its accommodation to and encouragement of human development. We know that all development proceeds with qualitative changes from fusion through differentiation to integration, and since people at any level of sophistication can use the golden rule, there must be varied ways to apply it as one matures.

Following Gilligan's work (2016) on the development of the ethic of care, I will illustrate three levels of maturation: the concrete first level; the second, differentiated level and the third, integrated or principled level.

At the most basic level, following the golden rule amounts to using projection. This would be good for me, so it must be good for you. It's easy to make light of this – it was even the basis for a cartoon character, General Bullmoose, who went around insisting that what's good for General Bullmoose is good for the nation. In fact, if you think the golden rule only applies at this level, you may not hold it in much esteem, as if it were a simplistic adage for children trying to get along with each other. Or even an easily misused rationalization for imposing one's own preferences on others. Indeed it is much more and better than that, as its current revaluing in the realm of philosophy attests (Wattles, 1996).

At a more sophisticated level, that of differentiation, we can think of people as full individuals. Here the golden rule supports discovering that what is good for me might be unacceptable to you and vice versa. For instance, the obedience I believe stifles autonomy may be a sign of devotion and intimacy to you. One way to think about the developmental task of differentiation is that it allows the full appreciation of meaning, the understanding that the same experience may mean different things to different people and that this difference is not a matter of right or wrong, but of simple diversity.

This differentiated level of development requires focus on individuals, which can feel frustrating to people used to considering abstraction or generalization as the goals of intellectual work. Yet even someone who finds great satisfaction in understanding differences, will eventually move to the third level, because awareness and acceptance of our differences in what I am calling stage two help press us toward resolving conflicts in a principled way, integrating experiences beyond their existing differences. For example, we may come to understand that respect is more important, and unifying, than any specific action or communication.

Since the right circumstances can throw us back to earlier developmental stages, any one of us might find ourselves at any of these levels, even if it is not where we usually function. A strength arising from the applicability of the golden rule at every level of development is that I can come to my group at any level of regression and still benefit. Here are examples of what I am calling the levels of development.

As an example of the first or concrete level, one practitioner arrived at Balint group spitting mad and in turmoil. He presented a conflict with a patient with lots of indignant self-justification. When the group worked on what he might be feeling, he was visibly moved. He participated at group's end in a much more peaceful way, saying little about the patient but expressing gratitude that others could understand his upheaval. This person really could not think beyond himself at the time of the group. Nonetheless, the Balint group work calmed him down and made him more able to think, not just to react. He could trust his group to show him compassion in his regressed state, and they in turn knew him well enough to trust he could mostly function at a more highly developed level.

From a more mature perspective another presenter was upset because despite her extra care of a laboring patient, the new mother was threatening legal complaints about her birthing experience. Over the course of the Balint group the physician grew more appreciative of having offered sophisticated technical medicine when the patient cared more about being able to have her friends and family in the room. Appreciating their differences helped her to relax and gave her mental space to reassess what had seemed like an unbridgeable gulf. The presenter grew calm enough to make a home visit to the mother and she eventually reported to her group that the conflicts resolved.

Finally, at the third or principled level, the hospitalist in a multi-cultural setting presented a situation involving a young patient, parents who would not discuss the situation and frantically frustrated staff. While the physician had handled the various issues well, he could not stop thinking about it. His Balint group was able to offer possible understandings of each of the very different participants. These included suggestions about the presenting doctor himself. People speculated he might be haunted by his wish to relieve the emotional pain of each one of those involved, as if this were the true meaning of palliative care. On rejoining the group discussion he announced he had resolved to do a grand rounds based on the case to help everyone, including him. Others might learn from it and he would address his now-conscious wish to care for all.

His work in the original consulting situation showed clearly how accepting this doctor could be of differences among people. In fact the staff had one religious approach to their work which conflicted with the different religion of the parents. The presenter did not get embroiled in this difference but found enough common ground to ease the situation. He acknowledged having treated people effectively. Yet this did not bring him peace until he was able to imagine generating understanding beyond the immediate needs, approaching universality rather than attending to individual details.

Each person in these examples benefitted from different aspects of the Balint work. They were able to do so in part because there was no right answer, no explicit or implicit requirement that a new view of the case be adopted. The very lack of didactic and conclusory material in a session makes the process uniquely well suited to apply to diverse developmental needs within the members. Because the leaders tolerate the frustration of not prescribing, the participants are free to discover and apply their own medicine.

The happy coincidence of Balint group structure and the golden rule has several ethical results including the reintroduction of wholesome caring into an unconstructive relationship without any overt reference to ethics. We can understand this ethical potency and its quality of implicitness, if we consider that a Balint group gives you practice in giving attention to another, giving attention to yourself and considering the mix of both, an opportunity for the tacit application of the golden rule as it fits you and your own ethical beliefs.

The parallels between Balint work and the golden rule might be only an interesting source of depth and strength for the method, but for the fact that practicing the rule leads to development. This means one long-term benefit from membership in an ongoing Balint group is ethical maturation. As Wattles (1996) explains: "Whoever practices the golden rule opens himself or herself to a process of change. Letting go of self to identify with a single other individual….one allows a subtle and gradual transformation to proceed…." p. 189 "The golden rule asserts the equal value of self and other; but it takes progressive self-realization to discover how great that value is. " p. 180 "The rule is an expression of human kinship, the most fundamental truth underlying morality." p. 188

Through habitual attention to all people in a relationship the members develop spiritually, so that prolonged Balint group membership supports the growth of greater equanimity and the maturation of one's judgment. We know a diverse Balint group may allow increased healthy emotional engagement in one's work. Now we see how it may do more.

More modestly Balint himself (1972) thought the exposure to different styles of doctoring had a maturing effect on one's professional self. "The discussion of *various* [emphasis added] individual methods, the demonstration of their advantages and limitations, encourages [the group member] to experiment…Every such experiment means a step towards greater freedom and improved skill." p. 306 His description of greater freedom and improved skill as fruits of diversity evokes the characteristic qualities of full maturity: flexibility, creativity and integrity.

My favorite benefit of Balint groups is reducing isolation, which I understand to occur at many different levels. After all, isolation of practitioners occurs naturally: confidentiality leaves us with fewer people to talk to; practice requires technical language, including diagnostic terms and other terms of art which pull us out of touch with our own and others' experiencing selves; and practice relationships may be conflicted and hard: we build them with people who tend to be in trouble or stressed or in pain.

The Balint group is designed to focus on these hard relationships, using everyday language, with folks who can understand what is meaningful about them. Because the structure and goals of the group parallel aspects of the golden rule, it is also able to bridge wide differences in religion or spirituality and to help us work our way nearer to each other. Because the practice of applying its processes and foci pushes us to develop spiritually, to a place where "the kinship of humanity is evident," the Balint group helps us grow nearer to the sacred without having to part from our traditions.

## References
Balint, M. (1972). The doctor, his patient and the illness, revised edition. International Universities Press: New York.
Chamorro-Premuzic, T. (2017). Does diversity actually increase creativity? In Harvard Business Review. Retrieved from the Internet on July 21, 2023:
https://hbr.org/2017/06/does-diversity-actually-increase-creativity
Gilligan, C. (2016). In a different voice. Cambridge: Harvard University Press.

Knowlton, E.K. (2017). Practicalities of diversity in a Balint society. Proceedings of the 20th International Balint Federation Congress, 123-128.

Sternlieb, J.L. (2018). Demystifying Balint culture and its impact: an autoethnographic analysis. International Journal of Psychiatry in Medicine, 53(1-2), pp. 39-46.

Wattles, J. (1996). The golden rule. Oxford University Press: New York & Oxford.

# 1.2   From Psychopathy to Compassion

Christian Linclau
Family Doctor (GP)
Walcourt, Belgium
doclinclau@gmail.com

## Abstract

To understand compassion with a detour through psychopathology and its neuronal mechanisms? How can a Balint group lead health professionals to compassion? That's what this paper proposes to explore.

How do we become able to understand others and to have compassion for them?

Do Balint groups offer tools to cultivate these qualities?

It occurred to me that it could be helpful to take a detour via psychopathy where there is no way for compassion and for others!

Maybe you already know the story of Phineas Cage? His case was described in 1848 by Doctor Harlow. This young man of 25 years old was a construction foreman for the railroad in Vermont, USA. He had a severe accident in which a large iron rod was driven completely through his head, destroying much of his brain's left frontal lobe. Incredibly, he survived this awful injury and was still able to speak and work as well as ever! But then strange things were observed. Before that event, Phineas was considered as someone pleasant, respectful and helpful by his workmates. After this incident, he started to be aggressive, he didn't care so much about others, taking considerable risks concerning everybody including himself and against the advice of his boss and friends. He started to lie and disregard everyone.

Later, in 1990, Damasio and Anderson [1] published the story of a woman who was involved in a road accident at the age of one and a half. She emerged alive and of course, it was a relief for her family! Everything went well until the age of three when she started to demonstrate bad behaviour like taking the toys of other children, biting them and being selfish. Punishments and remarks made no impact on her. She even ran away from school! Having been dismissed from many different jobs because of her poor conduct, she eventually ended up in a hospital at the age of 23 where she was diagnosed with orbitofrontal atrophy of the brain due to her very early accident.

These are the first steps to comprehending the link between the frontal part of our brain and socialisation!

To reinforce these findings concerning the link between the orbitofrontal lobe and the understanding and compassion for others, I cite another study [2]. In jail, one can find between 10 to 25% of psychopaths. Prisoners, generally speaking, have their orbitofrontal cortex reduced on an average of 22.3%. It's an atrophy without any injury (at least known injury!).

The uncinate beam is the neuronal wiring which allows the information to circulate from the orbitofrontal cortex to the amygdala at a high speed. This last is a part of the limbic brain which is the core of our emotions. The major role of the frontal cortex is inhibition. Michael Craig [3] and his team have emphasised that in incarcerated psychopaths, their uncinate beam was damaged. The consequence for these people is that their cortex is incapable of regulating their immediate impulsiveness for aggressive behaviour.

Nowadays, mental skills controlled by the frontal cortex are referred to as "executive functions". We can summarise these executive functions in 3 abilities:

1. The ability to control and inhibit actions: for example, to prevent an inappropriate gesture.
2. The capability to plan something, including a very distant goal in the future.
3. The skill of flexibility, enabling to adopt singular strategy taking into account different possible patterns of a specific work.

As a result, we can deduce that when there is a dysfunction in the orbitofrontal cortex, we probably will:
1. Consider ourselves superior to others, with an oversized ego, nothing slowing down our impulse or ability to reconsider our thoughts and behaviour,
2. Manipulate, deceive, lie to somebody just for our own benefit,
3. Be deprived of sensitivity, punishment having no impact on us. We could treat our neighbour as an object, with neither empathy nor compassion; socialisation would be impossible, but we wouldn't mind!
4. Act immediately, without taking consequence into account. Incapable of flexibility, we would hate unexpectedness.

Together, these four points are the symptoms of psychopathy.

We probably all know someone who is able to keep a straight face while telling a lie! Cerebral imaging [4] has shown that in that case, their orbitofrontal zone is switched off, making them believe their own story! This is helpful for our ego, isn't it? One could object: "not me, I'm not that kind of person!" Be careful: a survey [5] concerning our ability to drive has demonstrated that 80% consider themselves to be better drivers than their fellow-citizens…

Is it possible to limit this impact? Does any training exist? Spontaneously we might all be psychopaths! How is it possible to raise our children differently?

It seems clear that a child must know that they are not allowed to take a toy from another little one without their consent, they must take them into account and give it back! It's also obvious that an infant should seek approval from their parents and avoid their displeasure. Nevertheless, a warm and safe home environment and clearly defined boundaries must be present to enable the child to adopt a respectful behaviour. Traditionally, it's on the shoulders of the mother but the relationship within the couple is also extremely important (importance of the third)! It's now easier to understand that these conditions are not a reality for everyone and that the premise of the connections with others is already compromised for them!

To function adequately, the uncinate beam needs respectful education for our offspring, it requires us to be concerned about their future. The respect, the compassion for the stranger come from a warm and containing atmosphere between the limbic brain and the orbitofrontal cortex. There is an ongoing dialogue between the aggressive pulsion, the desire to possess, to have the power on one hand and the consequences for the future on the other hand. For example: when we hurt someone and then someone close to us tells us off, our amygdala will be blocked for a moment by our orbitofrontal cortex. This connects our mirror neurons which are the keys for mimicry learning. These mirror neurons are established in the pre-motor zone. They make us "embodied" with what's going on with the person we are facing, like sadness, stress, humiliation…these emotions, back to the amygdala, make us "feel" what the other could endure. The frontal cortex is now able to take another way with the other. As everything circulates so quickly, we are not conscious of that real storm of information and the contradiction in our brain! It requires flexibility and creativity to come up with identification of our "victim." Again, this is only possible if the circuit is well functioning.

Therefore, this complex wheel demands the involvement of all our cognitive capacities to work correctly. We have to train it like an athlete, exercising it regularly to perform! That means constancy, warming, learning from our mistakes, perseverance, and stretching.

Let's now have a look at our health professionals. Is compassion obvious in their behaviour?

Balint [6] proposes that we pay attention to a particular and complex concept he named "apostolic function". It means *"it's as if the doctor has the indisputable knowledge of what a patient is allowed to expect or not"*. In a way, it's something positive making the work of the health professional "endurable". There is also a dark side of this assertion: according to Balint, *it's the doctor's personality and* (almost) *only it which determine what's the right answer for any patient in front of him, no matter how different this person is*! What about listening to the patient which is so important in a care relationship?

If we go ahead, we could see a caricature of behaviour:
1. The doctor could feel superior, no place for doubt,
2. Twist the reality to convince the patient to follow his advice,
3. Not taking the other's specific condition into account,
4. Acting immediately.

It's not far from the four points we've seen above concerning psychopathy, is it?

That's when Balint came up with an interesting proposal: *make the health professional aware of his/her apostolic function and to step aside and think if it's helpful here, in this case or not...*

The Balint point of view is that we don't have to abandon completely our apostolic function while taking part in a Balint group; but to have just a minimal change which is already considerable!

To permit this "minimal" change, we need to train intensively the "driving belt" between the different parts of our brain as in sport. This work leads us to improve our compassion, creativity, acceptance of unforeseen situations, phronesis as John Muench [7] explained to us in the previous conference in Brussels...

How does it work in a Balint group?

The group will function like a catalyst of the prefrontal lobe. Indeed, when the presenter tells the story of his case, it's a first stop. A second stop arrives when he has to stay silent and listen to the group discussion. As with the child, clearly defined boundaries, the confidentiality, the non-judgment, the kindness of the group is necessary to offer the essential security. It's the main task of the leaders! Feelings circulate between the members of the group. The frontal lobe is then able to release is block and the hidden emotion can emerge through the mirror neurons. This doesn't happen necessarily immediately but from the back and forth through the free associations of the group. Therefore, the uncinate beam can make links between emotions and understanding of the case and to test what's good or less good in this situation. Sometimes, at a first look, the work doesn't seem to be helpful to the presenter, nevertheless, the different parts of his brain have been activated and something becomes possible: compassion is attained. Another important point is that it works also for the other members of the group (as well as for the leaders!). Even if the small discrepancy described by Balint is not observable there is already a considerable progress!

Balint also made another observation: the emotion felt by the health professional is often similar to the one the patient feels. As a result, it could be useful for the professional to get through their own perception to help this person. That means that the more caregivers know themselves and their reactions and tolerate them, the easier it is to be open to others, the more they can understand this "stranger" and accept their pain. A psychopath is obviously not able to do this.

The group is a major asset because you are not alone, it's less difficult to handle the fear, the unforeseen, not predictable facts. It's a parallel process to mothering, thanks to the setting and the leaders! This was absent from a psychopath's childhood.

As I said before, it's important to regularly exercise to be beneficial. It requires constancy, a warmup, perseverance and stretching. If we export these recommendations to Balint groups, it seems that once a month could be a good pace, avoiding absence to limit the consequences on the other members as well as for us and to enrich everybody with more interactions. Involvement of 3 years seems to be a minimum in order to be fruitful.

Creating a welcoming environment and incorporating a warm-up exchange at the start of each session—such as casual conversation—can set a positive tone and foster a rapport among participants. Sometimes it might be necessary to allow more time when something is too painful. Leaders must be willing and brave enough to slow down the process, even to stop it to avoid hurting the presenter, to being too intrusive. People have to finish the group without bowing their heads. Stretching could take place in the warmup and cultivate a confident atmosphere within the group, preparing the next meeting.

We are facing a positive spiral: the more different hypotheses are proposed by the group, the more they feed the presenter's internal circuits as well as those of the other members. The more they interact with each other, the more contradictions arise while brotherly cooperation make flexibility possible. Instead of a unique point of view, the group can construct a beautiful and coherent kaleidoscope. Where you can find the psychopath limited by his rigid pulsion from his ego, here we have the wonderful fertility of the group from which can be born a lot of possibilities, freedom, oxygen, life!

Life is the only way to have doubts about your certainties or maybe it's the contrary: to doubt your certainties is the only way to be alive!

When people exercise regularly, they continue to move throughout their entire life. I believe that care professionals who have been involved in a Balint group are still practising mutual aid and compassion!

## References
0. S. Bohler, *"Human Psycho"*, essay, Editions Bouquins, Paris, 2022. Reference who inspired this lecture … among others.

1.  S.W. Anderson and al., *"Impairment of social and moral behaviour related to early damage in human prefrontal cortex"*, Nature Neuroscience, vol. 2,1999, p. 1032-1037.
2.  Y. Yang and al., *"Volume reduction in prefrontal gray matter in unsuccessful criminal psychopaths"*, Biological Psychiatry, vol. 57, 2005, p. 1103-1108.
3.  M.C. Craig and al., *"Altered connections on the road to psychopathy"*, Molecular Psychiatry, vol. 14, 2009, p. 946-953.
4.  J.S. Beer and al., *"Exaggerated positivity in self-evaluation: a social neuroscience approach to reconciling the role of self-esteem protection and cognitive bias"*, Social and Personality Psychology compass, vol. 8, 2014, p. 583-594, and Y. Mao and al., *"Reduced frontal cortex thickness and cortical volume associated with pathological narcissism"*, Neuroscience, vol. 328, 2016, p. 50-57.
5.  O. Svenson, *"Are we all less risky and more skilful than our fellow drivers?"*, Acta psychologica, vol. 47, 1981, p. 143-148.
6.  M. Balint, *"The doctor, his patient and the illness."*, Churchill Livingstone, 1957, updated 1964, chapter 16-17.
7.  J. Muench, *"Proceedings; Balint core values: cohesion and flexibility"*, International Balint Congress, Brussels 2022, p. 87-94.

# 1.3 Cultivating Understanding and Compassion through Balint Work: An Opportunity to Promote Ethical Thinking in Everyday Work

Leonie Sullivan

Training and Supervising Psychoanalyst, International Psychoanalytical Association & Australian Psychoanalytical Society

Sydney, Australia

lesull@me.com

## Abstract

My paper focuses on a common thread, based on offering "a classic Balint group" across a variety of settings. The area of additional relevance and interest to be described, is that of enactment and its relationship in promoting a culture of ethical thinking as part of everyday work in health care. In providing an opportunity for participants to develop from the usual Balint membership, another aspect of the work has been noticed as a potential benefit. This comes from the experience of seeing oneself from the outside and others from the inside, which can address blind spots as well as leading to cultivating understanding and compassion for oneself, patients, and colleagues. This can promote thinking ethically in day-to-day work.

### INTRODUCTION

I work as an International Psychoanalytic Association (IPA) psychoanalyst both in Australia and the Asia Pacific Region. I am also an accredited Balint Leader with the Australian and New Zealand Balint Society. I am in private practice, so the Balint work I do is on a consultancy basis. This experience has provided me with an opportunity to affirm the effectiveness of Balint Work with family doctors, psychotherapists, psychiatrists, medical educators and students, psychoanalysts, psychoanalytic candidates, oncologists, paediatric staff, physicians, and mental health staff such as perinatal staff. Clinicians from China, Central Asia, Taiwan, Japan, India, France, USA, New Zealand,

and Australia have all provided feedback. Using the classic Balint method, in over 1,500 presentations, all had dilemmas involving inevitable enactments, where over and under identifications were played out within the presentation itself and work of the group.

This paper is based on my clinical and teaching experience in the Asia Pacific region and as former chair of training for both The Australian Psychoanalytical Society and The NSW Institute for Psycho Analytic Psychotherapy. I also chaired the ethics committee after having been a member for many years.

## BACKGROUND LINKING BALINT WORK TO ETHICAL THINKING
I worked for a period of 20 years as a member of a liaison psychiatry team at a large teaching hospital, where my role was to run groups, including Balint Groups. In hindsight this led to my conviction that ongoing Balint group work added a low cost and easily accessible method to promote a culture of interest in ethical thinking in everyday work as well as self-care. Group members were given the opportunity to present a dilemma about a relationship with a patient that they found challenging or wanted another perspective about. As a group leader, this experience helped me value the importance of a space to learn from struggling to understand and sit with uncertainty. Group members also recognised that all clinicians have blind spots. For group members, having a place in a group made room for the relationship between clinician and patient to be thought about in an alive way, free from the pressure to formulate, treat, or problem solve. Taking pressure off the "I don't know what to do about Mrs. B" where often the mutual helplessness and frustration was the last thing that was considered.

More recently, from feedback in both long term as well as the one-off intensive week/day experiences, participants describe the value of experientially coming to understand "the inevitable enactment" component in their work with patients. For example, one participant commented on what he called "a de-shaming" of his struggling with a specific cultural difference as a foreign doctor now based in rural Australia. As a group member sitting out of the discussion and experiencing the group's overwhelming frustration with the patient helped the doctor to articulate some of his own responses and so "re-find" his professional role. Initially the presenter was shocked at the strong response to his woman patient. He said that with the help of the group he was able to listen in a different way. Such comments point to ordinary Balint work being an achievable tool to promote a space in service provision for thinking about ethical/technical dilemmas. The observing self is known as having a capacity for reflective function. I want to stress that this is not the main aim of offering a Balint group but an additional benefit of the work.

## ETHICS AND ENACTMENT
As a long-term member of an ethics committee, I discovered firsthand how hard it was to interest people in the subject of ethics unless something was going wrong. Most hospitals and trainings and professional societies have ethical guidelines with ongoing

membership being conditional on a maintaining of what is termed "continual professional development". Despite this, serious ethical breaches continue to erode trust in our profession and damage emotionally vulnerable people and their families. Something extra is needed! Worldwide, most professional bodies list their ethical code on their website. This will often reflect professional and cultural differences. These are important in there being a frame or underpinning of professional competence. One of the concepts that unifies most ethical codes of conduct and practice is the notion "Above all do no harm."

From experience, few people look at these organisational codes unless something goes wrong. They are often dismissed as boring or not relevant to the pressure of everyday work. This can become a part of the organisational climate or culture. There are often extensive written guidelines online or on paper, which is where they stay until there is a problem. By group culture I am referring to both formal and informal structures, where members share a set of similar beliefs which then impact on the organisation. This is because "correct behaviour," hierarchical status, and certain rituals become established as the unique culture of a particular organisation. This can have serious adverse effects in terms of group culture and transmission of organisational difficulties. For instance, it is not uncommon to hear a presenter reflect about a wish to pass on a challenging patient to a more junior staff member because "that's how I was trained."

## ENACTMENTS
Stern (2009) comments on the role of mutual enactment as being an inability for both clinician and patient to mentalize an experience. An ordinary Balint Group offers the opportunity to attend to such situations by putting into words the experience of taking the presented case on. In the parallel process in a safely conducted Balint Group, it is common for this process of enactment to unfold in the group process until words are found and the experience shared. The group unconsciously reenacts the dynamics of the case. This is one of the reasons that training for Balint Group Leaders is essential so that the group can work safely with this process.

## MY BALINT WORK
In reviewing the last 12 years of my own Balint work, I have noticed that in the offering of the Balint Method to a variety of clinicians from different professional and cultural backgrounds, a common thread, benefit, or side effect emerged. This often resulted in group members reporting at the next meeting an increase in their capacity to be more comfortable with their own discomfort and so make better use of their relationships with patients.

The reflective capacity of any health professional can be impacted on by some patients. Becoming aware of this and having this understood in a Balint group can help any clinician develop a different perspective on themselves and their patient. In such cases, having a group mind to focus on the specifics of each clinician's story can make the difference in them being able to bear their experience long enough to emotionally digest the experience and speak about it.

## ENID AND MICHAEL BALINT

Originally, Enid and Michael Balint helped to identify and further work with "blind spots in the clinician," thus helping all of us to this day "bear the burden of helping the patient enough." The Balints described the style in which people are expected to face challenges of being able to think and relate to illness, pain, death, and the ways the helping professions use their technical skill and knowledge. This conception can influence the way in which the clinician not only talks to the patient and relates to them; it also impacts on the way in which the clinician expects to be treated by the patient. This is often outside of conscious awareness.

A clinician who for some reason is intolerant may be drawn into being dismissive. The case that stands out is that of a doctor who had refused to see a terminally ill patient because of the patient's expression of angry feelings. He was aware that someone else might have been more prepared to listen to the patient's struggle with being given a terminal diagnosis. He stated he did not have the capacity to listen and unpack the pain the patient was in. He wanted to send the patient to a more junior member of staff. The patient, a hospital orderly, was shocked by his diagnosis and that he was given so little attention, since in his work he had always gone that bit extra to help. These things were explored in the group. The group was so full of the story they also reacted in a similar way, which shocked the presenter a lot. The group members agreed that this wasn't a case! It was an ongoing group, so the emotional parallels were not lost but utilized in the work.

Some of these attitudes are not always in the clinician's awareness, nor are some of the attitudes that the patients have towards their treating clinician. Something in the relationship remains unmentalized. It is an awareness of this dimension that I believe helps prevent the more serious boundary violations that are at the extreme end of the continuum of enactment behavior. Developing such awareness is often only possible with the introduction of a third position. This is why in many Balint groups the person presenting hands over the story of the patient and themselves to the group to work on while they remain out of the discussion.

In 1993 Enid Balint discussed the need that all clinicians must make an imaginative identification with the patient. She described the clinician as being engaged in a balancing act: both needing to "enter into" the patients' painful experience (even when this is disorganizing or painful) and at the same time struggling to not to lose sight of their role and function as a clinician. If the clinician is emotionally present, it may become apparent that the patient, just by being themselves, will unwittingly attempt to draw the clinician into some sort of re-enactment of painful past relationships. Enid Balint wrote about the bi-phasic nature of empathy, as a part of the mental activity of the clinician in being aware of the pull to be drawn out of the therapeutic role and then refinding it.

## ENACTMENT THEORY AND LINKS TO BALINT WORK

Others have further elaborated the challenges posed by enactments and the importance of any clinician being able to be aware of how they are perceived by their patients, for example the work of Mitrani (2001). Some expectations and perceptions are hard to take or be aware of, for instance, if the clinician has a blind spot because of their own situation. The research work of Peter Fonagy (2002) has highlighted the importance of "thinking about thinking." He acknowledges the origins of some of his ideas to the Psychoanalyst Wilfred Bion (1962) on Reverie and the concept of the Container - Contained. Fonagy and Bateman (1995) claim that the mentalizing stance requires the clinician to own their unique anti-mentalizing errors.

Steiner's (2000) paper on containment, enactment and communication is relevant as it names the process of a psychic retreat as a type of enactment. A recognition of the role enacted can advance the understanding of the nature of the retreat and underlying organisation of the personality.

## LANGUAGE AND ENACTMENT

Steiner noted that "language can only lead to proper communication if the clinician attends not simply to their patient's words but to their context and to the non-verbal cues that accompany them. It is now equally clear that clinicians must attend to their own reactions, to the countertransference in the broadest sense, and this includes not just their emotional state but also their thoughts and actions."

Internal conflicts in the patient and clinician can become externalised in the work of the group and elements from both internal worlds can even be played out as the group works. Feelings and associations are created in the group and can lead to a pull of being drawn to actions. Any clinician may find themself playing a role ascribed to them by the patient. The possibility for further thinking emerges if the clinician can contain their propensity for action. The support and experience in the group gives an opportunity to look at the pressures put on the clinician and the feelings aroused in the group, which are a part of the situation that needs to be understood. In a Balint group, reverie can be restored when the presenter experiences the group working with the story or case. By this I mean the presenters imaginative capacity to make links between the emotional reality in the room and themselves and the patient.

The British psychoanalyst Betty Joseph in her 2003 paper 'Ethics and Enactment' assumes some kind of enactment with patients is inevitable. Her point is that all clinicians are impacted by what they see and hear in the consulting room. It is when we are not aware of these feelings that as clinicians, we can be pulled towards living them out or enacting them.

The point she makes connects to my focus on Balint work and its link to helping with ethical thinking in everyday work, not just when something goes wrong. The provision of a regular well-conducted Balint group provides a space to examine the huge "grey area" as described by Joseph (2003). The "grey area" leads to questions of when does an ordinary enactment move towards a breach of ethical behavior? The Balint process in its focus on the relationship between practitioner and patient will so often keep the principle of "do no harm" alive, long after the group session is over. It provides an opportunity for group members to make use of their group experience when they return to their consulting rooms. Patrick Casement (1992) refers to a similar process, as "the internal supervisor." In feedback, group members often refer to what was said in the group helping them think differently about challenging situations.

Joseph highlights a few issues, including clinicians' unconscious need to give way to or enact their own defensive needs, as being an insidious problem. This can influence the way we talk, our tone, or simply laughing at a joke, all of which whether conscious or not keep things comfortable between patient and clinician. She cautions about the way negative feelings are sometimes dealt with, by being drawn into our own or patient's evasions and hence not facing up to the emotional reality of what is really going on in the consultation.

## CONCLUSION

When Patrick Casement talks about a process of the acquisition of an internal supervisor, he is referring to a capacity for reflective functioning. In a Balint Group the members of ongoing groups report a similar process of internalizing and being supported in their thinking capacity (especially around enactments) by the group's mind. Thus, Balint Groups provide a simple and low-cost method to keep ethical thinking both interesting and constantly alive in everyday clinical work. I am looking to create a more formal pilot study to further document this. The method has produced positive outcomes across theoretical, professional, and cultural differences. This is due in part to the work being done by the group, as it is facilitated to understand a clinical dilemma rather than provide a solution in response to it. Once further understanding is gained the relationship between patient and clinician benefits from a fresh perspective.

## REFERENCES

Balint, E. (1969) The possibilities of patient centered medicine. J.R. Coll.Gen.Pract.17(82):269-276.

Balint, E. (1993) The doctor the patient and the group revisited. Routledge. London.

Bion W.R. 1962, Learning from Experience. Heineman. London.

Bateman, A & Holmes, J. (1995) "Introduction to Psychoanalysis, Contemporary Theory and Practice. Routledge. London.

Casement, P. (1992) On Learning from the Patient. Guilford press New York.

Fonagy, P. et al. (2002) "Affect Regulation, Mentalization, and the Development of the Self." Other Press, New York.

Joseph, B. (2003) Ethics and Enactment. European Psychoanalytical Federation (EPF) Conference.

Mitrani, J. (2001) Taking the transference: Some technical implications in three papers by Bion. Int.J. Psychoanal.82. (6) 1085-1104.

Steiner, J. (2000) Containment, Enactment and Communication. Int.J. Psychoanal. 81. 245-255.

Stern, D (2009) Partners in Thought: Working with Unformulated Experience, Disassociation, and Enactment. Routledge. New York.

# Chapter 2

# 2.1 To Intervene or Not Intervene, That Is the Question

Albert Lichtenstein PhD, LMFT
Guthrie Clinic, Weight Loss Center
Sayre, Pennsylvania, USA
albert.lichtenstein@guthrie.org

## Abstract

Deciding when and how to intervene in a Balint group as a Balint group leader is often complex and at times difficult to teach. Interventions determine not only the frame of a Balint group but also the safety and richness of the content and learning. This paper will discuss what can be called "non-discretionary" interventions that need to be made in order to make a Balint group a Balint group, "discretionary" interventions that lead to increased understanding of the case but may for various reasons go unspoken, and a process for how a leader might make a decision to intervene.

I have noticed over time that many interventions that occur to me while leading a Balint group go unspoken. This has led me to try to delineate my basis for choosing to make an intervention and what my cognitive process is when a possible intervention occurs to me. How well thought out is this process and why is it that some interventions just feel right? In this presentation, I will examine these questions.

In 2006 Marian Lustig and I wrote about how Balint groups help integrate intuition and reasoning in medical decision-making building on Daniel Kahneman's work (Lichtenstein and Lustig 2006). Kahneman (2003) described two cognitive systems that operate with decision making: system 1, or *intuition*; and system 2, or *reasoning*. Intuition is fast, parallel, automatic, effortless, associative, and emotional. Whereas reasoning is slow, serial, controlled, effortful, rule-governed, flexible, and neutral. With experience, proficiency, and increasing mastery, care providers, and Balint leaders, can begin to use automatic intuitive processes to make decisions. This presentation will incorporate this way of viewing decision making into understanding Balint leadership.

Leading a Balint group requires multitasking: listening to the case content while monitoring and directing group process, tracking time, tracking group development, and monitoring one's own emotional reactions, to name some of the tasks (Johnson et al 2004).

Over time, and with experience, some of this becomes an automatic, intuitive process which allows interventions to bubble up. There are times when I can articulate the rationale for an intervention – sometimes in real time, sometimes after they are in my head demanding to be released. Since the group is happening in real time, there is time pressure to decide whether to intervene or not. Not all interventions will or should be spoken. Given the time pressure and complexity, an accurate intuitive, automatic system can help. However, when an intervention pops into my head do I trust my intuition and judgment or don't I?

I have begun to categorize interventions as either non-discretionary or discretionary. In my training in the American Balint culture I would classify non-discretionary interventions as those that are necessary to promote basic group functioning. If these interventions are not made, the group process will suffer and the group may not feel adequately held by the leaders. Examples are those interventions listed below that maintain basic group structure, frame, and safety.

> Most all structural interventions (when using push back)
>> Calling for the case
>> Asking for questions of fact and limiting the questions to facts
>> Suggesting the presenter rest
>> Inviting the group to 'take' the case
>> Providing enough time for the group to discuss the case
>> Bringing the presenter back in
>> Ending the group
> Keeping the frame
>> Starting and ending the group on time
>> Keeping intrusions out
>> Redirecting tangents to their relevance to the case
>> Keeping to one case and presenter's viewpoint if multiple group members know the patient
> Safety
>> Limiting critical questioning or comments
>> Limiting group members pushing others, especially the presenter for self- disclosure
>> Limiting focus on the presenter's psychological dynamics
>> Helping group members take responsibility for their own thoughts
> and feelings

With some "non-discretionary" interventions it is clear from the structure of the Balint method, or architecture as Sternlieb (2011) called it, that it is the role of the leader to direct the group process. With other "non-discretionary" interventions when the frame or group safety is in danger of being violated, a Balint red light goes off and the need for intervention is clear. Intuitive, automatic reactions serve well in those situations. The primary caveat is thinking about how to phrase those interventions in order not to shame a member or the group. With practice that also becomes more automatic.

Discretionary interventions are interventions that enrich the group's understanding of the case, emotional reactions, and relationship issues. The group will function simply fine without these interventions, but the depth of understanding might suffer. Examples of reasons for discretionary interventions are as follows:

> Balancing representation of the provider and patient
> Commenting on the emotional tenor of the case or group discussion
> Reminding the group about the presenter's dilemma and words in the presentation to focus the group
> Highlighting metaphors
> Deciding whether to allow for colleague or supervisor relationships as the central element of a case
> Breaking or allowing silence
> Balancing participation by group members

"Discretionary" interventions may, or may not, optimize the richness and understanding that come from the case presentation and discussion. Klein (2003) describes intuitive functioning as depending on accurate pattern recognition. Data is perceived from multiple inputs in a holistic format which leads to the ability to make rapid judgments. However, a range of variables increase the salience of information used for intuitive judgments, not the least of which are 'hot' states of high emotional and motivational arousal (Kahneman 2003). How do I know if my thinking is a product of the case and the needs of the group or my own emotional reaction coming from somewhere else?

To function optimally, a Balint leader needs to be sufficiently self-aware to monitor use of the intuitive system, have some sense when emotional reactions are playing a part in the situation, and to know when to slow down and effectively bring the reasoning system into action. Novack et al (1999) called this 'reflection-in-action'.

When an intervention comes into consciousness, hopefully it brings the reasoning system to the fore. Ideally the function of the reasoning system is to monitor the use of intuition and deliberately override a quick, typically used but inaccurate response. However, the corrective operations of the 'reasoning system' may be impaired by such factors as time pressure, concurrent involvement in a different cognitive task, 'morning people' performing the task in the evening, 'evening people' performing the task in the morning, or even by being in a good mood.

Since it is certainly quite possible for a well-functioning group to have a fruitful group with minimal intervention, as I consider this dilemma, I have certain questions somewhere in mind that help determine whether to make a discretionary intervention.

Is the group working well without me?
Does the group need to develop a sense of its own agency?
How important is the intervention to the understanding of the case?
Is the intervention for me or for the group?
Early in the group – will the group get there on its own?
Late in the group – is there time for the group to change focus?
Is one member so totally dominating or the group using that member to the detriment of process?
Will a group member relate some introduction of personal information or another case to the case presented?
Does a little advice giving from a member help that group member get involved?
Is this silence helpful or not?
Has enough time elapsed for my co-leader's intervention to have played out?
Is support with calm presence enough or does the group need more?

When I think of an intervention, I cannot say I go through those questions systematically. The consideration of those questions has become relatively automatic. I usually repeat the intervention to myself a couple of times to see how it sounds and whether it makes sense. Borrell-Carrio et al (2004) describe the process of diagnosis and treatment as creating a clinical tension which is heightened by uncertainty and relieved with the acceptance of a diagnosis and plan. This tension can be difficult to live with and lead to premature closure or over reliance on intuitive automatic processes. Even though I feel less anxious leading a Balint group than I did early on, it is common when I lead Balint groups to feel the same tension with uncertainty. Hopefully, the uncertainty is helpful in calling on the reasoning system if it is not paralyzing.

Here is a case example that illustrates a number of leader processes I have identified in this paper.

A member of our Balint group presented a case of a patient she saw in training years ago. The memory of the patient had stayed with her. The patient had died by suicide sometime after the presenter had moved on in training and stopped seeing them. The relationship had been a good one and the patient had seemed to be improving.

We were using the pushback method in this group and all the non-discretionary structural interventions such as asking for a case, asking for clarifying questions, pushing the presenter back, and bringing them back in were all used.

Several discretionary interventions occurred to me around the themes of abandonment, guilt, and boundaries. I made one early intervention "Why does this patient stick with us" in hopes of getting to some of those issues. The group responded to that intervention with the pain and responsibility that might be felt. I had thought of the intervention "Why is this patient always punctual and showing up to clinic often?" The group discussed this without my input. That indicated to me that at least I was tracking the group reasonably well. Later in the group it occurred to me that the presenter was probably the same age as the patient's daughter. I decided it was too late in the group to get to that and in the remaining moments the group went back to a sense of guilt, remorse, fear for such patients, which was more useful than my intervention might have been at that point given that the group continued to work actively and to deal with genuine feelings. That proved to me once again that sometimes a non-intervention is the best one.

In the case cited above my co-leader and I discussed many of the unspoken interventions in the debrief in the hopes of learning from them. In fact, we thought of interventions that might have been brilliant had we actually thought of them in real time. Something that seems to happen quite frequently.

As in other tasks, the more experience one gets as a Balint leader, the more comfortable one becomes with trusting one's intuition. Preparing this presentation has helped me to gain some understanding about the mystery of why an unspoken leader intervention is never spoken. Over the past 30 years of leading Balint groups I have come to trust my intuition and go with it a fair amount. After all, the group can choose to ignore an intervention if it does not fit or come back to the intervention when they are ready. Very few interventions are damaging to the group unless they are mean spirited or shaming, or repeatedly over-controlling. I have come to feel the necessity of intervening in non-discretionary situations, and the virtue of questioning whether to intervene in situations that I believe are discretionary. Hopefully, I get it right. And if not, my co-leader is sure to let me know.

## References

Borrell-Carrio, F. Epstein, RM. Preventing Errors in Clinical Practice: A Call for Self-Awareness. Annals of Family Medicine 2004;2(4): 310 -316.

Johnson, AH, Nease, DE, Milberg, LC, Addison, RB. Essential Characteristics of Effective Balint Group Leadership. Family Medicine 2000; 36(4): 253 -259

Kahneman, D. A Perspective on Judgment and Choice: Mapping Bounded Rationality. American Psychologist 2003;58(9):697-720.

Klein, G. (2003) Intuition at Work. Doubleday: New York.

Lichtenstein and Lustig. Integrating intuition and reasoning--how Balint groups can help medical decision making. Australian family physician (2006) vol. 35 (12) pp. 987-9

Novak, DH, Epstein, RM, Paulsen, RH. Toward Creating Physician- Healers: Fostering Medical Students' Self-awareness, Personal Growth, and Well – Being. Academic Medicine 1999; 5 (May): 516- 520

Sternlieb, J. Balint Group Architecture, <u>Journal of the Balint Society</u>, Vol. 39 p. 17-19, 2011

*A previous version of this paper was presented in absentia at the Russian Balint Society Congress in St Petersburg, April of 2022.*

*I am indebted to Jeff Sternlieb for his thoughtful editorial comments for this paper.*

# 2.2   May We Speak of the Dead?

Andrew Leggett MBBS, MPhil (UQ), PhD (Griffith)
Clinical Director, Mental Health Alcohol and Other Drugs
Services, Mackay Hospital and Health Services, Queensland
Health
Mackay, Queensland, Australia
Andrew.Leggett@health.qld.gov.au or eruditescribe@gmail.com

## Abstract

This paper offers the experience of a meeting of a Balint clinical reflection group for psychiatry registrars training in a regional city in Queensland, Australia, a meeting in which the leader accepted the offer of a case of a patient who died, in spite of the leader's prior knowledge of a tradition of reluctance to accept such cases. The author, in asking, 'May we speak of the dead?' invites discussion of this question.

**May we speak of the dead?**
In the author's experience of Balint clinical reflection work, in intensive workshop groups led by accredited Balint leaders, he has encountered a reluctance to accept cases where the patient has died. The reasons given for this prohibition focussed on the lack of a continuing doctor patient relationship, one in which it would be possible for the doctor to gain from the group insights into the nature of the relationship with the patient which would enable enhanced understanding to be carried into the next consultation. If the patient has died, there can be no continuing relationship, there will be no next consultation, so why discuss the case in a Balint group?

The theme of the 23rd International Balint Federation Congress, in Boulder, Colorado, USA, 'Cultivating Compassion and Understanding Through Balint,' invites discussion of how we might 'transform our thinking about creating meaningful professional relationships' (American Balint Society, 2023). Among the situations, regarding which papers are invited, is the question of failure, failure of the group. This paper opens a question beyond that of failure of the group. It asks whether or not the leader failed when he accepted a case for discussion of the presenter's sense of failure when a patient has died, especially as the death was considered as a consequence of failure of the work of the presenter and colleagues who strove to prevent this death, a death which was a consequence of addiction. This paper includes an account of a Balint group's effort to respond compassionately to that sense of failure.

Kerri Sackville (2019), in an article entitled 'Why is it still so taboo to speak ill of the dead?' argues that 'the most obvious reason to respect the dead is our compassion for the grieving.' Given that the doctor who offers the case of a patient who died may be grieving, and may be supporting other clinicians or family of the patient who has died, should we consider the Balint group a potentially safe space for the compassionate support of the grief process of the doctor, in the interests of the doctor, and of the relationships with the living that the doctor continues to hold a duty to sustain?

This question arises in the setting of a monthly Balint Clinical Reflection Group for psychiatry registrars working in the Mental Health Alcohol and Other Drugs Services of the Mackay Hospital and Health Service in a regional coastal town in north Queensland, Australia. The author identifies himself as the leader of that group. The paper has been circulated among members of the group for comment and revised accordingly prior to submission.

After the call for a case, there was silence. Perhaps thirty seconds pass before a participant said that he hadn't prepared a case. The leader reassured the group that there was no need to prepare in advance: the case could be any of any recent consultation with a patient, especially those that have the doctor feeling curios, trouble, puzzled, worried, including those that come to mind only when the leader calls for a case.

Then there was another long silence. Another participant said that, if no one else has a case, he has something. The leader invited him to go ahead.

The presenter told the group that the case troubled him because he was called about the patient when he was a way at a conference, just about to present a paper. The manager of the service in which he worked with patients suffering addictions was calling to inform him that the patient had died after injecting a cocktail of drugs, including something laced with fentanyl.

As the presenter began to tell the story, the leader reflected on what he had previously been taught in supervision, not to accept cases of patient who have died, because the discussion cannot contribute to improving the quality of on an ongoing doctor-patient relationship. In spite of this, the leader decided to accept the case after checking with the presenter that he had experienced an ongoing treating relationship with the patient. The leader made this decision after noticing that the presenter was visibly distressed. The leader thought to himself: *Isn't this was Balint is for—to address the emotional and psychological aspects of the doctor-patient relationship? What could be more important in that sphere, and more distressing for a trainee psychiatrist than to struggle in processing the loss of a patient through sudden death?'* The leader checked with the group, who were unanimous that the case should be accepted. Then he invited the presenter to continue.

The presenter described his initial reaction to the news of the death as being one of worry that he had failed the patient, that he had missed something. Then he reflected that he had been told the pathologist report revealed that patient had been found deceased with the tourniquet still on his arm and his injecting kit beside him. Then he shifted to speaking of how warmly he had felt towards the patient at the last consultation. The man had a young family and was in the process of establishing a business that was succeeding. He had been optimistic, proud of a year's abstinence from intravenous drug use and in the process of gradual reduction of methadone towards cessation, which was only a couple of steps away. The presenter spoke of his disappointment that the patient had lapsed, but denied feeling angry about it, just sad. Sad, but disappointed. He spoke about himself and the other clinicians in his team liking the patient and had taken pride in having supported to patient through his recovery, almost to the point of cessation of treatment. It had been a shock to learn of this sudden death of a patient who had been doing well. The presenter than spoke of feeling guilty for being away at a conference, proud of his achievement in having a paper chosen for presentation, but guilty that he wasn't at work at home, supporting the rest of his team through the bereavement. He then thought of how devastating the loss would be for the patient's wife and son. What would it be like for the little boy to grow up without a father? The presenter remembered talking with the patient about the pleasure he experienced playing with his son, and the plans he had of things to share with his son in the future.

The presenter then paused. The leader waited for him to continue, but he did not, so the leader opened the case for questions from the group. There were none, so the leader invited the presenter to mentally push himself back from the group and observe, reminding the group to speak of the presenter and the patient, but not to address questions to the presenter while he was pushed back from the discussion. The leader than invited the group to discussion of the case.

After a few moments silence, a participant acknowledged how distressing it must have been for the presenter to hear this news while he was away at the conference, when his last experience of the patient had been so positive, with such cause to be hopeful and optimistic.

The group was smaller than at previous meetings, with some of the participants called away to do urgent patient assessments, in spite of the meeting being scheduled in designated protected educational time. Although every member of the group spoke at some stage during the meeting, the leader found himself more conscious than usual of the silences between speeches. He felt pressure to fill them. Most comments focussed on the perspective of the presenter—how sad and how disappointed he must feel that someone he had thought was doing so well lapsed and that lapse was fatal. One participant spoke of difficulty comprehending what the preschool age son would make of the loss of his father. Other spoke empathically of the painful loss the boy's mother was imagined to have experienced.

Well into the meeting, after a long silence, the leader commented on how the perspectives of the presenter, the patient's partner, the patient's son had all been addressed. Then he said: 'I wonder what the patient might say to us if he could speak, if he could hear us?'

One participant said, 'I think he would be embarrassed and express shame. He would be disappointed in himself and tell us he was sorry. He didn't mean to die. He just wanted to have some fun. He had been good for so long.' There were more comments to the effect that he might say he was angry with himself for lapsing; angry that the drugs he had bought had been contaminated; that he hadn't thought about the risk; that he had scored on impulse. Participants were adamant that he had not meant to kill himself. There were comments about how worried he would be for his wife and his son; how much he would want his son to remember him as a father who worked hard and didn't do drugs; how much he regretted not being around to watch his son grow up, take him to the park, teach him to kick a ball, play cricket, take him to swimming lessons. Another participant commented that we don't know what happens when we die, but if there is any existence after death, she imagined that the patient might feel relief at being in a peaceful place now where he no longer had to struggle against his addiction: that it might be a relief to be dead.

It seemed that the intervention regarding what the patient might say to the group if he could speak redirected the focus to the patient's perspective and functioned to free up the group to work together more fluently. After a period of such fluency, there was a long silence. At this point, with about twelve minutes of the meeting remaining, the leader invited the presenter to rejoin the discussion with the group.

The presenter said that he valued the discussion, especially the comments about the difficulty of losing a patient who had been doing so well. He spoke further about how, on return from the conference, he had supported his clinical team, who were taking the loss very hard. While at the conference, he found it difficult to adjust to the fact that he could not be with them when they received the bad news. He agreed with the group's view that the patient had not been trying to kill himself. Rather, he thought the lapse had been impulsive, triggered by some reminder or some chance meeting, perhaps even due to boredom with sobriety. 'Maybe,' said the presenter, 'he had thought *just one more time*. We can't know, but if he was still around, in some form, and able to look on at us and at his son, he would be wishing he could say sorry, and would be very sad at not being there for his son.'

The group took up various aspects of this, with similar comments. Soon it was time to finish. The leader thanked the presenter and the group, then reminded them of the next meeting, in a month's time.

So, in Balint group meetings, may we speak of the dead? On this occasion, the leader decided to accept such a case. This paper invites discussion. within the international Balint clinical reflection community, of the merits or otherwise of such a decision.

### References
American Balint Society (2023) *Call For Papers 23rd International Balint Federation Congress, in Boulder, Colorado, USA, 'Cultivating Compassion and Understanding Through Balint'.*
Sackville, K. (2019) 'Why is it still so taboo to speak ill of the dead?' *The Sydney Morning Herald*, 6 May 2019, downloaded from the internet 12 August 2023: https://www.smh.com.au/lifestyle/life-and-relationships/why-is-it-still-so-taboo-to-speak-ill-of-the-dead-20190304-p511o9.html

# 2.3   Balint Work in Times of National Trauma:
# Caring for Oneself in Order to Care for Another as Portrayed in a Verbatim of a Zoom Balint Group in Israel after October 2023

Shai Krontal
Family Physician and Psychotherapist
krontal@gmail.com

Daniella Cohen
Clinical and Educational Psychologist and Organizational Consultant
codan29@gmail.com

## Abstract

We describe a Zoom Balint group in times of war that began after the largest terrorist attack Israel has experienced, one that is still considered a national trauma.

On October 7, 2023 at 06:30, the entire nation of Israel awoke to sirens, as thousands of missiles were fired upon us. Hamas launched a premeditated and brutal attack on dozens of Kibbutzim, villages and cities and on the participants of a music festival, killing 1,200 men, women, and children, and abducting over 200 into Gaza.

This was and still is a national trauma for Israelis, expressed in fear, depression and decreased functioning. After the events of October 7th (known as "the Black Sabbath"), war broke out.

The authors have always been committed to the idea of living alongside our enemies, and empathize with the suffering of the people in Gaza. Beyond the collective trauma, we are both personally affected, as described later.

The authors have led a Balint group on a bi-weekly basis for nine years. Its participants, professionals from a multitude of fields, have joined at different times.

We will describe our understanding of Balint groups at times of collective trauma, specifically addressing the following points:

- Leading a trauma-adapted Balint group: attention to unique trauma-related content and processes;
- "A Wall Falls Down" in Balint as both doctor and patient become vulnerable: an analytical term referring to the symmetry forced on a doctor-patient relationship when are both influenced by the same intimidating external events;
- The Balint group creates cohesion and belonging, allowing the resumption of a routine where we deal with the relationship between doctor and patient, kicking off the trauma recovery process and warding off the threat of disintegration.

-

On the day war broke out, we updated each other after a missile fell in our neighborhood. Daniella felt strongly that the group should convene as usual; the collapse of trust and chaos around us demanded it. We proposed this to our participants, but they declined as they were too busy protecting themselves and their families.

We convened for the first time, 2 weeks after October 7th, on Zoom. Instead of presenting a case, the participants were asked to share their personal and professional experiences of war. This was an advance decision as part of a trauma-adapted understanding that one cannot deal with the doctor-patient relationship before treating the doctor. We also used this method during COVID-19. After sharing, the participants asked *us* how we were doing, we responded and Shai talked about his brother's family, who were trapped in the safe room as terrorists wandered through their home in a kibbutz near Gaza.

The next meeting, presented here today, occurred a month after October 7th, also via Zoom.

The meeting began with a siren. We all ran to our respective shelters, and after 10 minutes the meeting resumed. After sharing the siren experience, we requested and received the participants' consent to record the meeting.

Daniella begins the meeting, addressing Shai and asking everyone to share how they feel at this difficult time, how their families cope and how their professional roles are affected, and whether they would like to present a case later. Out of sensitivity to ongoing trauma, we avoid the regular prompt for a case, offering the option to get there gradually.

The group is silent.

Daniella addresses Shai again, suggesting that self-disclosure is effective in emergencies, and relates how she met families with children in the stairwell when the siren sounded, and how worried she is for her family which lives a few blocks away. She shares that her daughter-in-law is alone with the children, as their father has been drafted for reserve duty. She could only come back to the Zoom session after hearing they were safe in a shelter.

*Addressing Shai again emphasizes the infrastructure of our shared leadership, which stabilizes the ability to work in a group, when our national security systems have failed us. Beyond the effectiveness of self-disclosure, Daniella points out the "wall falls down" principle, reminding everyone that the leaders also share the terrible experience of the current reality, there is a symmetry between them and the participants, in order to encourage the return of the internal thinking and observation that is characteristic of Balint work.*

G. is a dentist at a hospital who has been with the group for two years. He is first and describes his decision to hospitalize a patient with pus-draining necrosis because she is from a city under fire.

Shai invites more participants to share.

*Although we are aware of the consequences of stopping someone who begins to present a case, it felt important to "sacrifice" G for the process of the group.*

R, a director of social work at a hospital, continues:

> I'm on high adrenaline, when I need to slow down in a meeting with a patient. It's harder to be fully attentive, even my breathing has changed. It's hard for me to make time for the group, but I'm here.

The group is silent.

*Apparently the silence helps everyone breathe and enables the next participant to talk about the terrible things that happened to her family.*

P. is a geriatric specialist. Her close family lives in a kibbutz near Gaza and were under fire in the safe room on October 7th. One family member died.

> The day before yesterday I was in Eilat, where my family has been evacuated along with their kibbutz. I saw them now after a month, they're okay. What stands out is the conversation - as if it was yesterday, not like a month has passed, behaviors of disorder and chaos and... sadness... I'm lucky there's work.

*We observe traumatic content in R's words about physical experiences, and in P.'s, which describe a feeling of altered time perception.*

The group is silent.

B. is an RN and veteran participant. Both her sons are conscripted to combat service and four of her daughter's close friends were murdered at the music festival.

> At work, I also have a conscripted team. The workload suits me, it's a source of sanity. Two patients in the department are involved, one's children were evacuated to Eilat and a woman whose sister and niece were kidnapped.- a cloud of sadness enveloping…

N. is a pediatrician whose nephew was injured at the beginning of the war. She's been a member of the group since its inception.

> I'm a full-time grandmother now, as the kindergartens don't have missile protection. It helps because I have very deep questions, so it's a bit of a relief from work. At work, I have almost nothing. There are three new anorexics.

*The leaders, who are attentive to the trauma, notice the preoccupation with questions of morality and ethics and anxiety about the future.*

Daniella suggests that N present the cases but N prefers not to because she is not yet sufficiently familiar with them.

*We previously heard about a pus draining and now we hear that the group is reluctant to deal with the trauma of what reportedly happened to women's bodies.*

> Shai: If anyone who hasn't spoken yet wants to speak they are welcome.

Y. is a psychiatrist. One son of his is in the army, and the second, who has special needs, is at home as his hostel has been closed down because of the war. Y. joined the group one year ago and leads a Balint group at his hospital.

> I feel very tired. I sleep more and I'm still tired. The state of mind that changes from 'business-like' and maniformic is quite terrible and going down to the shelter with patients is something…

*This is reminder of the "fallen wall" between doctor and patient.*

A. is a Ukrainian-born GP who has previously reported the effects of the Russia-Ukraine war on him and his family. His niece escaped the music festival after seeing atrocities.

He is the last to speak and talks at length about his situation and a conscripted son who is not in danger.

> Just a few days ago, someone came to me at the clinic, after hours, he said 'if you can still see me, maybe we can talk'.

> Daniella: Go ahead, go ahead…

He describes a long-time patient of his, a 39-year old heterosexual single male who has been discharged from military service – in a unit that was not his organic unit - because of anxiety. He received anti-anxiety medication in service, and was now asking to extend the treatment. A. describes his deliberation on whether to prescribe sedatives, contrary to trauma treatment guidelines.

> He hasn't had a relationship for a long time. I talked to him in the past about late singleness, he is good looking, modest, an accountant… He has no family, a strained relationship with his parents. He began to fall apart in his reserve unit. He says: 'I tried but I couldn't function.' And he was released from his position with a sense of shame and panic attacks. He said it was probably related to being alone. 'The drugs you gave me really help me, it bothers me that I couldn't cope alone.' I gave him Clonazepam, I felt it was what I needed to do… And then he asked for more of the drugs I gave him… Maybe it's less of a Balint question but more medical, I don't know…

*A's question of whether the case is suitable sounds like another part of the collapse of all the truths in our environment.*

> Daniella: It is a Balint case and it doesn't matter if we call it Balint, we have time to address it… (to the group) Do you have any informative questions?

*Consistently with trauma treatment, Daniella offers containment and the leaders identify that the group is ready to transition from personal stories to a case, and Daniella's intervention, asking for informative questions, is a return of the setting, where the outside rules have collapsed.*

> G: Did you give him more?
> No, I told him he had a few more pills for this week… I asked him about suicidal thoughts, and he said he doesn't plan to die. He was such a hero, he did reserve duty until the age of 39, and he did it well, he was respected, and he respected himself, and now at the end he said, 'I just couldn't handle it, so they released me.'

> Shai: It's an informative question, but it also marks the beginning of the discussion. A, take a few steps back, we'll be with your case. Can you handle being outside the discussion?

*This is a classic Balint intervention and a trauma-adapted addition that examines the ability to be alone.*

> A: Sure.

The group is silent, then the first response comes from the psychiatrist.

> In the question of the therapeutic treatment, that is talked about a lot, but as doctors, we don't have good drugs for all this trauma. It illustrates how terrible it is… There are many things that we can't really help.

A few other participants talk about medication and helplessness. Short silence.

*Identifying trauma related helplessness.*

> Daniella: How do you feel about the emotions A described in his case?

*The leaders' referral to emotion is well-known in Balint work, in states of trauma we encourage the discussion of a routine and control, and here we emphasize the Balint routine which returns us from defensive talk and steers us towards the emotional experience.*

N. the pediatrician:

> Confusion. I feel like I'm not qualified enough to help, and I don't know if this person will become psychotic.

*We note the traumatic experience that threatens to break down (psychosis) and the change from potency to impotence.*

> Daniella: A. talked about a 39-year-old man, alone, without a relationship, alone.

> Y: The presentation wandered between referring to the very personal matter of this person, to a person who is immersed in trauma where the person is no longer important.

> N: The family doctor serves as a support circle for a person with no support.

After the participant points out the important role of the doctor in supporting the lone patient, an association comes up, presented randomly, but it will change the understanding of the case.

> P: A little off-topic, but I spoke with a senior officer about all the terrible killings, he told me that on the first day, there were three suicides of very senior

people, including one physician, and my thought was: "how could they do this to us? How could they add more deaths?"

Shai: So maybe the Clonazepam is what the *doctor* needs?

The group is silent.

Daniella: The story here is about loss. I can remember another terrible period in Jerusalem, it was close to me and my son was injured in a terrorist attack. I worked with a psychiatrist who attended those attacked and evacuated to the emergency room by touching their hands as a means of healing.

A particularly long silence.

Shai: A, if it's convenient for you, you can be with us in the few remaining minutes.
A, the presenter: I asked him if he was under any direct risk. And there wasn't. The next day he praised me for understanding that, after his discharge, "I don't have anyone else to get tranquilizers from". I am the only one who will prescribe it.

Daniella: Maybe he wasn't alone for a moment.

A: Right, loneliness… He himself began to say that it probably also affects him and I also thought of myself, that I'm not alone in facing this. I'm talking about myself! Not about anyone else. I'm going through the period relatively easily. It actually gave me an understanding of similarity and difference, he's not injured, but he's hurt…

The meeting ends.

We have presented the story of a veteran Balint group that convenes in a time of war and national trauma to hear the participants' traumatic experiences and was able to deal with a Balint case only a month after war broke out. The case in point is a soldier who appealed to his GP for relief from his emotional anguish after being exposed to combat and released from duty. In the group discussion a free association came up about a doctor committing suicide on the first day of the war, helping us understand that doctors who are exposed to the external reality they share with patients may feel hurt and need emotional relief.

Our leadership focused on maintaining the group, which began with the sirens and personal stories with adaptation to the national trauma. There was also awareness and self-disclosure on our part. In these situations there is need for special attention to expressions of trauma. The self-disclosure made present the concept of the "Fallen wall" and enabled, through a reverse process from the leaders to the participants, the acknowledgement of the doctor's vulnerability. This was required so that we could provide the proper treatment for others' trauma.

Despite the difficulty in resuming the Balint routine, like any other routine disturbed by national trauma, we realized that our ability to return as leaders with adapted structuring of the Balint rules conveyed an important message of hope and trust and rehabilitation of thought processes, which is so necessary when thought itself is attacked – in patients and doctors alike.

The presenter's ability to return to the group and talk about the difference between himself and the patient and between "hurt" and "injured" is evidence that the return to Balint work under the conditions described, allows for the recovery of the mentalization processes essential to the restoration of the caregiver's role during national trauma, as well as for emotional relief.

# Exploring Ethical Dilemmas in Balint Groups:
## Workshop on the IBF Code of Ethics

Andre Matalon, GP in Israel, Vice President of IBF Board*
Tove Mathiesen, Psychiatrist in Denmark, President of IBF Board*

Balint groups serve as invaluable spaces for healthcare professionals to explore the emotional dimensions of their work, enhancing both clinical skills and containing ability. However, the ethical landscape within Balint groups warrants careful consideration to ensure that participants engage in meaningful, respectful, and ethically responsible interactions. A code of ethics is the essential core value of any society and is especially important in the helping professions, where relationships between people are a central issue for understanding, intervention, and research. A Code of Ethics for the International Balint Federation has been prepared and was presented at the last Council meeting in Stockholm in spring 2024; it has been sent to the different National societies; and it will be discussed in depth at this workshop.

Through experiential exercises and case discussions, participants will examine ethical dilemmas encountered in Balint group settings, how to address these, and what the role of the local Balint Society or the Ethical Committee or the IBF could be in such cases. We will discuss dilemmas arising around confidentiality and privacy concerns, informed consent procedures (using material from Balint groups without asking the participants), managing relationships in the group (such as romance between leaders and trainees), addressing power differentials among group members, and navigating cultural and diversity issues.

In a collaborative and reflective environment, this workshop aims to deepen participants' ethical awareness and competence, enabling them to engage in Balint group processes with integrity, empathy, and wisdom.

We hope that attendees will leave with a heightened ethical sensibility and a practical toolkit for applying ethical principles in their Balint group facilitation or leadership. The board would like to offer those interested the opportunity to participate in the Ethical Committee of the IBF to be formed after the conference.

* Both have been part of the editing process around writing the Code of Ethics.

# Chapter 3

# 3.1 Professional 'Siblings' in Balint Groups

Yuval Shorer, MD

Psychiatric Department, Soroka Medical Center

Faculty of Health Sciences, Ben Gurion University of the Negev

Beer Sheva, Israel

yuvalshorer@gmail.com

## Abstract

Balint groups convene colleagues from the numerous care professions. Themes and emotions brought in Balint groups raise the hypothesis that perhaps the connections we have are stronger than mere colleagues and rather more like the relationship among professional 'siblings'. The article echoes "Freud's Blind Spot" stating that: "more than parents, more than educators, more than friends, or lovers and pets, our brothers/sisters shape us 'to be who we are'. Through discussing Balint group vignettes and leaders' discussions we try to show that group interactions could echo sibling transference that influences group process and leaders' cooperation.

## Introduction

Balint groups often include colleagues from different health care professions. At one of our Balint Group Leaders conferences, the leaders in the opening circle raised the question of our needs when we come to Balint. Some declared a desire to learn, others to seek mutual enrichment by working together in the same 'professional house'. An experienced family doctor Ruhama, a newcomer to Balint, enquired humorously "would you adopt me into your Balint family?". In another leaders' conference a family physician pondered "why do mental health professionals come to Balint? Family doctors obviously benefit from Balint, but don't mental health people have their own groups?!"

At another conference, the topic was "Who or what are we protecting in Balint groups?" There was an open and honest talk about maintaining boundaries, keeping to Balint rules, leaders looking after each other and protecting the presenter as well as maintaining safety and preserving the organization where they work and more.

Towards the end of the discussion somebody suddenly raised the question as to the important responsibility we had for each other in the group. We were struck by the thought that perhaps the connection we have is stronger than mere colleagues and rather more like the relationship among professional 'siblings'.

Elisa Albert, in her book "Freud's Blind Spot" (1), claimed that "more than parents, more than educators, more than friends, or lovers and pets, our **brothers/sisters** shape us 'to be who we are'". As a young child, Freud was greatly influenced by the birth and sudden death of his younger brother Julius. Julius was born when his brother was 17 months old and died 5 months later. In a letter to one of his confidantes Freud confessed "I welcomed my younger brother with malice and true infantile jealousy, his death left the seed of guilt in me". However, Freud ignored the importance of siblings in the case descriptions he wrote.

If indeed we could consider each other professional 'siblings' then how does the integration of different professions affect the process within the group? We will discuss this through examples from Balint groups.

**Case 1: Patient "number one"**

In the Balint group the day after the opening discussions in the leaders' conference, Ruhama who was mentioned above, hastened to declare "I want to introduce my 'patient number one'". Emotionally, she continued "I want to share with you the treatment of my father. You can see that I have been in the profession for a while, I am now approaching retirement. I am an only child and accompanied my father on his cancer battle for two years at the end of his life. I felt that I had to save him and so I did everything I possibly could for him. I took advantage of the connections I had in the hospital, but in the end, nothing helped and he passed away. I am left with feelings of guilt that I didn't do enough for him".

A heavy silence hung in the group. The participants looked at each other uneasily. They were ambivalent, torn between identifying with the presenter and following Balint rules. The story was moving but the dilemma existed – how should we deal with it?

The participants then shared stories of dealing with their own parent's illnesses and their participation was very intimate and open:

Yosef, an internist: "I remember how I was informed in the middle of a conference abroad about the illness of my father, who had been hospitalized. I was really torn between continuing with the conference or returning to Israel".

Rachel, a gynecologist: "I remember what it was like when my father was sick and I attended to him. It doesn't leave me to this day".

The leaders looked at each other but said nothing. There was an atmosphere of a shared fate and empathic identification within the group. Suddenly one of the veteran members commented with frustration "I feel very alone in the group this time. I planned to share the treatment of a very special patient of mine. He was not my father, but rather a patient at the clinic who reminded me of issues related to my father RIP. Yes, I too lost my father under difficult circumstances, of which some of you know, because most of us have known each other for a while as veteran Balint members. However, somehow in the group today I don't feel comfortable talking about it".

The group was in a dilemma – should they continue sharing their personal experiences or not? It did not seem appropriate to stop the process, seeing as it had already begun. It was evident that the sibling identification with the presenter was so strong that the Balint rules, not to deal with personal issues, had been forgotten. This process had flooded one of the participants with memories that he did not want to share with the group. Who should the leaders protect? The presenter? The participant who did not talk? Or the group as a whole?

Later, in analyzing the leading process, the leaders shared that it had been their first group to lead together. In hindsight, it could be that they should have deliberated openly with the group whether it was appropriate to present this case at a Balint group, whether they should have stopped the presenter and discovered the nature of the case before it was presented or to stop her as soon as it became obvious that it was a personal story from her private life.

The memory of the sharing in the opening circle of the conference, when all the 'professional siblings' met was surely fresh in their minds and perhaps it affected both the group leaders and the participants. Had the participants felt like the presenter's siblings and protected her in a kind of shared fate of 'professional siblings', even at the expense of deviating from Balint rules? Should the leaders, like parents in the family, protect the participants who shared their similar child-parent dilemmas? Or should the rules have been followed – the group is not meant to be a therapy group? How should they, in a Balint group, have dealt with the emotions of the participant who protested?

Should this group, which was a one-time group, have established clearer boundaries for the discussion? It is perhaps worth noting that when a group is well established and has met over a period of years, there can sometimes be room to present a personal case.

**Case 2: The lost sister**

A social worker presents a dilemma at the Balint group (led by two mental health professionals): "I am part of an inter-professional treatment team in a psychiatric day hospital. I take care of a 19-year-old girl who has been in the hospital for two years, due to a mental breakdown accompanied by prolonged functional decline. At the beginning of the hospitalization, it was thought that she was suffering from schizophrenia. Later it became evident that she had been sexually assaulted in the family. She reacted in states of dissociation, as well as repeated suicide threats. I am her case manager. The team, which consists of psychologists and psychiatrists, now wants to release the patient from day hospitalization. However, I feel an emotional commitment to her and am afraid of suicide attempts and that she won't manage well outside".

In this group, the clarifying questions phase was longer than usual, as is often the case when the case is one of sexual abuse. In the group process, the members shared situations in which it had been difficult to protect a patient.

The mental health professionals seemed to understand the complexity of the case and sympathized with the dilemma of the social worker. They understood that she felt like a parent who needed to take care of their child. Many questions were asked, such as: Are we sometimes overprotective? When do we know that a patient can be trusted? Do we sometimes not give the patient a chance to grow?

The leaders noticed that the family physicians were relatively quiet in the group and asked why that might be. The latter shared that they do not often treat this type of patient and felt that they had less to contribute from their professional experience.

Towards the end there was a request from one of the family doctors to share "something personal that is not easy." The leaders noted that there was not much time until the end of the meeting, but nevertheless gave a chance, recognizing that the family doctors up until then had spoken little. The doctor then shared that, as a young girl, she had witnessed her sister's suicide and had been left with a deep sense of failure. She described that it had been a very difficult experience that shaped her personal life and later also her professional life as a doctor. Everyone felt great empathy for the doctor's pain.

The leaders were in a dilemma, whether to allow the group to respond to such a painful emotional experience a few minutes before the end of the meeting. In the end, they did allow the discussion to continue. However, after a short period of sharing in the group the leaders stopped and explained that it was a topic that required more processing than the remaining time allowed for.

After the meeting the facilitators felt that an opportunity had been missed and spoke with the participant briefly. They were concerned that she would be upset after bringing up a distressing topic that was not satisfactorily dealt with. She admitted that she did feel let down.

The emotional sharing in the group, and the nature of the case presented, caused us to once again ponder: Can we think of Balint as a group where professional 'siblings' sit together to share dreams, fantasies, and professional dilemmas? Do the group leaders act as 'professional parents' from different professions? Among the professional 'siblings' there are differences in professional terminology, attitudes and knowledge. In addition, the participants have varying levels of knowledge and experience of participating in Balint or other groups. We all carry images of an ideal brother or the perfect sister. A large part of our lives as siblings is conducted in the space between these optimal images and the painful reality. Meeting in the group may cause painful issues from the past to rise, as happened here.

### Case 3: physical and emotional contact

In another group a family doctor introduced the case of a 55-year-old male with no family. He was a long-term patient of hers who was about to be released from an internal ward at the hospital to his home. He had been hospitalized to clarify various physical complaints, but no organic source was found. However, he continued to complain about non-specific pains and had asked the doctor to make a home visit because he "was having trouble leaving the house because of his pain". The doctors shared that she had debated whether to make a home visit, since no cause was found for his pain, and also because he was a strange man whose home was always in a state of neglect. Although she decided to comply with his request, during her visit his behavior was erratic, he did not get out of bed, refused to talk or answer questions and asked that she examine him physically. She hesitated, in the absence of an urgent indication for the need to do so.

The family doctor consulted with the group about how to proceed. Should she demand that the patient come to the clinic or comply with his requests for home visits? In the group it was apparent that although there was a desire to understand the 'somatic' patient in order to help the doctor understand her emotions, there was a lack of sufficient information. A long silence ensued in the group. To get out of the impasse, the leaders suggested that the group try to imagine what kind of person the patient was and his possible background. The group remained quiet. The leaders pointed out that perhaps the dilemma reflected the distance the doctor had felt in relation to her patient.

Dana (family doctor): I don't have to imagine; he reminds me of the appearance and behavior of a patient I treated in the past. He was unkempt and had a bad smell which made it difficult for me to examine and treat him.

Moshe (psychologist): I can visualize a person who has a criminal characteristic or had an abusive past and maybe the doctor sensed this.

Group leader: Fantasies are hypotheses that can be worked with in therapy to understand our patients and why we are at a standstill with them, as is done in mental health.

Shira (family doctor): But we are family doctors. We have to physically touch the patient to examine him, I am in close proximity to him, in his own house. That's hard for me. We don't work with fantasies!

There was frustration in the group as if there was hidden criticism of family doctors who were perhaps less experienced in dealing with uncertainty and relying on their imagination when treating patients.

After another long silence the group leader pointed out that perhaps this was a patient we refer to as "the rejected patient". He then asked what could make us feel rejection towards a patient.

The group shared stories of treating patients whose bodies look unpleasant or who have an unpleasant smell, in addition to situations where the patient hides information and presents complaints that are difficult for the doctor to understand. A silence ensued, which was broken by Rafi, a family doctor. "I am a family doctor, and my sister is a psychologist. When we meet, it is not always easy for us to share with each other the cases we treat, there is a distance between us. Each of us has difficulty describing exactly what we do when working with patients. Maybe it's something about touch, connection, a little bit like how I feel at this moment in the group."

A sense of relief was felt in the group, something had become clear. This case concerned the differences that exist between professional 'siblings' regarding the emotional and physical contact in a relationship with a complicated patient. Perhaps a hidden competition exists between professional 'siblings' to gain emotional insights in the group as well as feelings of anger and jealousy that are common among ordinary siblings.

In the parallel process, amongst the group of professional 'siblings' a split was created. On the one side were the 'good, understanding siblings' from the mental health field, who have a therapeutic imagination and emotional insights. On the other side were the 'difficult siblings', the family doctors, who stand at the forefront of treatment, do the hard work, are involved in close physical contact with the patient and sometimes find it difficult to openly share their feelings of disgust and rejection.

**Thoughts about parental-leadership aspects**

Sibling transference is not limited to the therapy room. It can contribute to family - like cooperation in groups with strangers especially when the environment symbolically duplicates a harmonious family atmosphere (2). Participants in a long-standing Balint Group may be emotionally involved with their "brother/sister" in the group, which may contribute to a positive familial atmosphere.

The case stories highlight the tangle of emotions and loyalties that exist in the relationships between professional 'siblings', especially when the case takes us on a journey to the threshold of our own homes and families.

The first case of a physician failing to save her father triggered in the group a kind of sibling identification which challenged the leaders. They were, in a sense, drawn into a parental over - protective countertransference. Perhaps the leaders, in having to decide whether the case was suitable for Balint Group discussion, were afraid to be thought of as "bad parents" in front of 'all-loving' siblings? Are cases of a physician failing to treat or save a close family member legitimate Balint cases?

In the second case a mental health dilemma in a group led by two mental health leaders might have drawn the professional siblings into an idealized parental transference in which they wanted to please the idealized parent/leaders? And as a consequence, did this lead them to miss the more 'troubled' sibling in the process?

In the third case, in a group led by two mental health practitioners, the discussion of a difficult somatic patient caused a split between mental health professionals and family physicians. Was the split a parallel process, or a competition between the preferred and the rejected siblings? The sharing in the group of a personal sibling issue helped to resolve the split in the group. Did the definition of the patient as "rejected " by one of the leaders stimulate the split in the group? Was there a different sibling transference to each of the two mental health leader-parents? And what influence did any rivalry have between the two mental health leader-parents?

Psychological concepts, myths and Jungian archetypes try to conceptualize the relationship between siblings (2). They range from twin fusion, admiration and idealization, jealousy, mutual dependence to hostile dependence or rejection (3).

Sibling and parental transference such as competition, jealousy, anger etc. are feelings we often 'keep to ourselves' in Balint groups and in life in general.

What a challenging territory to explore.

### References
1. Albert E. Freud's Blind Spot.p76 Free Press 2010.
2. Abramovitch H. Brothers and Sisters Myth and Reality. Texas A&M University Press College Station, Texas, USA, 2014. Hebrew version- Resling PUB, 2016.
3. Bank S., Kahn M. The Sibling Bond. New York: Basic Books,1981.

# 3.2 You Can Teach an Old Dog New Tricks:
# Balint in the Veterinary World

Shana O'Marra, DVM, DACVECC
Associate Professor, Washington State University School
of Veterinary Medicine
Pullman, Washington, USA
shana.omarra@gmail.com

Jillian Room, RN, LCSW
Private Practice
Portland, Oregon, USA
jillianromm@gmail.com

## Abstract

Similar to human medical care providers, veterinary medical practitioners navigate complex human relationships when providing care to pets. Veterinary professionals experience high levels of job-related stress and distress compared to other professions. The fee-for-service model and the dual role of pet owners as caretakers and decision-makers can contribute to moral distress, which has been also reported to be particularly pervasive among veterinary providers. This paper explores the application of Balint groups in addressing the challenges faced by veterinary professionals, focusing on the provider-patient-client relationship. The authors share their experience implementing Balint groups for veterinary professionals, both in-person and virtually, discussing the challenges and themes that emerged during the sessions. Cases presented in the Balint groups revolved around interpersonal conflict, role discomfort, and moral injuries. Based on the authors' experience, Balint groups are feasible in veterinary settings and are well-suited to address the challenges faced by veterinary professionals in their relationships with clients and patients.

Like many care providers, veterinary professionals experience job-related stress and distress. A recent review of literature examining veterinary well-being found a high prevalence of psychological stressors and increased risk of burnout, anxiety and depressive disorder in veterinarians compared to other occupational groups[1]. Significant psychological distress was documented among the veterinary workforce by the Merck Veterinary Wellbeing Study III[2], with 9.4% of veterinarians experiencing serious psychological distress as measured by the Kessler Psychological Distress Scale, a steady increase from prior reports in 2017 and 2019. Younger veterinarians <34 years old experience the highest rate of serious psychological distress (16.7%). Veterinary staff experience even higher rates of serious psychological distress (18.1%). Burnout is high among veterinarians and veterinary staff as measured by the Mayo Clinic Physician Well-Being Index, with 30.5% of veterinarians and 49.6% of veterinary staff experiencing high levels of burnout.

There is friction that is inherent to the practice of veterinary medicine in the United States of America. Most veterinary care exists in a fee for service model, introducing a dynamic of customer/salesperson into the provider-patient-client relationship, and magnifying societal issues of equity and access to care, especially when considering the beneficial effect of pet ownership on human health. The role of the pet owner is both the caretaker of the pet and the final authority and decision maker in a very explicit way, often involving financial considerations. In addition to financial friction, the legal status of pets as property is out of step with the value that most pet owners and veterinary practitioners place on the human animal bond. A recent survey by the Pew Research center found that in the United States of America 97% of Americans considering their pet a member of the family[3]. Further complicating the provider-patient-client relationship is the fact that most veterinary patients end their life with euthanasia being performed by a veterinarian rather than natural death. The natural lifespan of most pets is a fraction of a normal human lifespan, so it is common for veterinarians have multiple interactions with clients around death and dying. The death of a pet frequently uncovers unresolved emotions around loss of loved ones in both clients and providers.

Given these issues, it should be no surprise that moral distress is pervasive in veterinary medicine and figures prominently as a driver of burnout and psychological distress. In 2018, Moses et al[4] published a survey of veterinarians that introduced the concept of moral distress to a wide veterinary community. Over 70% of respondents reported experiencing moral distress. Of those respondents, 85% reported conflicts of opinion with clients over their pet's course of treatment as a source of moral distress.

With growing awareness of high rates of suicide[6] and psychological distress among veterinary professionals, professional well-being has become a prominent focus of professional organizations and scholarly activity in the veterinary world. Today, there are many options for crisis care, group support, and even some institutional changes to promote well-being. Although much progress has been made in recent years, most existing interventions in veterinary well-being primarily focus on individual repair and self-care, neglecting the crucial provider-patient-client relationship.

Research on interventions to prevent or mitigate moral distress in veterinary medicine is lacking, however qualitative research in human healthcare providers suggest that moral conflict does not lead inevitably to moral distress. Traudt et al[5] interviewed a cohort of human critical care nurses and found that despite working in an environment saturated with moral conflict, the majority of nurses did not experience the damaging effects of moral distress. Moral agency, moral imagination and moral community appeared to offer protection against moral distress. Balint groups offer a potential solution by creating a safe space for reflection. When cases fraught with moral conflict are brought to a Balint group, the process itself serves as an exercise in moral imagination. In grappling with the case, the group can serve as a moral community, perhaps allowing the presenter to gain awareness of and confidence in their own moral agency.

While under supervision by her group co-leader and credentialed Balint Group Leader, Jillian Romm, RN, LCSW, the author began offering a Balint Group to veterinary professionals in the Portland, Oregon area in the summer of 2019. Each Balint group was followed by a formal debriefing between the co-leaders. Case notes were kept by the leaders about the nature of the cases, challenges, and recurrent themes from the start of the group in July 2019 until January 2022.

Balint Group sessions were offered in-person initially, at an urban non-profit emergency and multispecialty animal hospital. Veterinarians and staff were invited to participate, and during the in-person phase of this group, an average of 8 participants joined, primarily from small animal general practices and the staff of the multi-specialty hospital. With the onset of the pandemic, the group transitioned to virtual meetings via Zoom platform. This transition led to participation from distant regions in the US, as well as to smaller sized groups, with rare repeat attendees. The authors focused on providing Balint for clinicians who had direct access to clients, and included veterinarians, veterinary nurses, client liaisons and support staff.

Implementation of Balint groups in the veterinary setting required addressing the provider-patient-client triad, rather than the traditional provider-patient dyad of human medicine. This approach parallels the Balint process for human medical providers with non-verbal patients. Composing the group of providers who have client contact allowed for discussions about the relationship between the veterinary professional and the client. This group was most useful for clinicians who had a relationship with the patient AND with the client, as it was within those relationships that most cases emerged.

Participants were prepared for the group with an explanation of structure adapted from American Balint Society materials[7], specifying that the relationship to be examined was the provider-patient-client relationship, with interventions from the leaders, to imagine what it is like to be the provider and the client in the relationship. Due to the open membership of the group, every group was preceded by a brief description of the process.

Balint Group discussions with veterinary colleagues were rich and dynamic, and appeared to meet the goals of the Balint process. Throughout the discussions, themes emerged within cases offered. Interpersonal conflict and role discomfort were common, with several cases resulting from client discussions about goals and costs of care. Several cases were presented in which providers were accused by the client of caring only about receiving payment for care despite the provider caring deeply for their patient.

Cases about the moral injuries of practicing veterinary clinicians elicited strong emotions and support from group members. Managing patients for whom the care is seen as futile, unnecessary, unhelpful, or painful for the patient, were common themes. Discussing these painful clinical scenarios lessened the isolation reported by many clinicians, while providing a vehicle for sadness and grief.

Grief and sadness were shared as common experiences throughout our cases, as is often the case in human medicine Balint groups. Multiple cases involving patients with no owner, or those in which the owner seemed disengaged with their pet were presented. Presenters often felt a close bond with the patient, standing in for an absent or uninvolved client. Group members often shared their attachment and love for their patients and identified with the animal, which the group recognized. The group reflected about attachment and recognized that this attachment may have complicated relationships with the client.

Participants readily explored the emotional content of the cases, but required intervention from leaders to reflect rather than simply observe. Interventions addressing the relationship with the client were made frequently by leaders, in attempts to open and clarify the relationships. Leaders tended to be active in these conversations, and to include questions and reflections about the relationships. The financial considerations and stressors of owning a professional practice and employing staff and colleagues frequently arose during our case discussions, brought forth by the cases offered.

An anonymous survey was circulated in June 2021 inquiring about participants' experience, ability and interest in attending future sessions. Respondents included four veterinary technicians, two client service professionals and one veterinarian. Ages ranged from 28–55 (median 40) years of age, and participants had a median of 16 years in the profession (range 3–30). Five participants had attended a virtual session and two had attended an in-person group. Although only seven prior group attendees offered feedback, there was agreement that they had developed new insights about their work, were able to consider aspects of cases that they had not previously considered and developed new insights about future work. Scheduling difficulties were noted as the most frequent reason for non-repeat attendance. All participants agreed or strongly agreed that they had "received new insights and ideas that will shape my own work in the future." In general, all responders noted they enjoyed working on the provider-patient-client-relationship.

Although the author's experience leading Balint Groups included only veterinary providers, she has also participated as a group member in multiple training intensives and an online group in which she was the sole veterinary provider among human medical practitioners. Those groups successfully engaged with the provider-patient-client triad in the author's case presentations and provided an incredibly supportive and insightful experience. Her positive initial experiences as a veterinarian among human medical providers led her to pursue additional training in the hopes of bringing Balint groups to a wider veterinary audience. In addition to her own experience, the author is aware of several efforts to engage veterinary professionals in Balint work.

Two veterinarians are currently undergoing fellowship training with the American Balint society and recently began offering an online group through the Veterinary Information Network, an online community for veterinarians.

A multidisciplinary group including veterinary faculty, athletic training faculty and faculty in the family medicine residency program at Washington State University was recently formed. The author attended the inaugural meeting of this group, and observed rapid accommodation for the differing patient populations and rich discussion among the participants.

Balint groups have proven to be a robust and adaptable structure to apply to varied provider-patient relationships. In the future, the author hopes to continue to spread awareness of and access to Balint groups for veterinary providers in private practice and academic environments as well as house officers and trainees.

## References

1. Pohl R, Botscharow J, Bockelmann I and Thielmann B. Stress and strain among veterinarians: a scoping review. Irish Veterinary Journal. 2022;75:15-38.
2. **Brakke consulting.** Merck Animal Health's Third Veterinarian Wellbeing Study Reveals Increased Health Challenges and Psychological Distress Among Veterinarians. Merck Veterinary Wellbeing Study III. 2022. https://www.merck-animal-health.com/blog/2022/01/18/merck-animal-healths-third-veterinarian-wellbeing-study-reveals-increased-healthchallenges-and-psychological-distress-among-veterinarians/

3.  "2023 Pew Research Center's American Trends Panel." Pew Research Center, Washington, D.C. (July 7, 2023) URL: https://www.pewresearch.org/short-reads/2023/07/07/about-half-us-of-pet-owners-say-their-pets-are-as-much-a-part-of-their family as a human-member/
4.  Moses L, Malowney MJ andWesley Boyd J. Ethical conflict and moral distress in veterinary practice: A survey of North American veterinarians. Journal of Veterinary Internal Medicine. 2018;32:2115-2122.
5.  Traudt T, Liaschenko J, Peden-McAlpine C. Moral Agency, Moral Imagination, and Moral Community: Antidotes to Moral Distress. J Clin Ethics. 2016 Fall;27(3):201-213. PMID: 27658275.
6.  da Silva CR, Gomes AAD, Dos Santos-Doni TR, Antonelli AC, Vieira RFDC, da Silva ARS. Suicide in veterinary medicine: A literature review. Vet World. 2023 Jun;16(6):1266-1276. doi: 10.14202/vetworld.2023.1266-1276. Epub 2023 Jun 8. PMID: 37577194; PMCID: PMC10421543.
7.  Balint Group Process. An Introduction to Balint Work. The American Balint Society;                                                                  2016. https://www.americanbalintsociety.org/content.aspx?page_id=86&club_id=4 45043

*Portions of this work have been previously presented at the American Balint Society National Meeting 2022 and published in the International Journal of Psychiatry in Medicine: O'Marra, S. K., & Romm, J. S. (2022). Balint in the Animal World: Balint Groups for Veterinary Professionals. 57(6), 521-526.*

# 3.3 All Creatures Great and Small:
## Cultivating Understanding of Human-Animal Relationships in Balint Work

Veerle Van Geenhoven, PD
Dr.phil.habil., M.vet med., M.A. Germ.ling.lit
Center for Clinical Veterinary Medicine
Munich, Germany
V.Geenhoven@lmu.de or VeerleVanGeenhover@t-online.de

## Abstract

How can doctors and therapists develop understanding of patients whose pets mean the world to them without falling into clichés? How can Balint work contribute to this task and cultivate understanding of cases, in which human-animal relationships appear to play a significant role, while standard Balint work is solely about relationships between humans? This paper promotes the integration of human-animal relationships into Balint work. First, I will show that when we acknowledge the common neurobiological denominator in human and animal emotions, human-animal relationships fit well into object relations theory. Next, I will offer some examples that illustrate how awareness of the presence and influence of animals in Balint cases can increase the potential for free associations and insightful perspectives.

## Introduction

This paper is about integrating human-animal relationships into Balint work, a challenge that I originally took up realizing that within veterinary medicine there is an urgent need for profession-related supervision [1,2,3]. Within this context, I was primarily occupied with the question of whether and how veterinary cases, in which obviously human-animal relationships are a central part, could become a substantial part of Balint work.

As it is common practice for pet owners to view their pets as family members [4], I soon realized that reflecting on human-animal relationships in Balint work need not be restricted to veterinary cases. That is, if a pet plays a significant role in a patient's life, there is no reason to remain silent about this relationship when this patient is brought in as a case during Balint work. In fact, human doctors and therapists reporting on a case often mention that the patient involved has a pet. This piece of information is rarely picked up in subsequent Balint work. This disregard may reflect the ambivalent ways society deals with pets and other animals. Also, it is in line with Roth's observation that "in the analytic literature, there is a subtle tendency to diminish the importance of human-pet relationships and accent the pathology of pet attachment [5:453]." He brings in clinical cases showing that transference and other psychodynamic processes take place within and through human-animal relationships. Hence, the psychodynamic potential of a patient's bond with a pet can become a valuable source in understanding a professional relationship with this patient.

To ensure that pet relationships are not overlooked in Balint work, it is helpful for those presenting an animal-related case or bringing in an association about a patient's pet — and for group leaders as well — to have some basic theoretical insights into the emotional life of animals [6]. Even among veterinarians, this knowledge is not an obvious part of their training. Research on the psychology of the human-animal bond (HAB), that is, on the question of what animals can contribute to the emotional life of their owners, and vice versa [7,8], demonstrates interest in its psychodynamic aspects [5,9]. A number of interpretations of the HAB stands in the broader tradition of object relations theory (ORT), ranging from Bowlby's attachment theory [10,11,12] to Klein's object relations approach [13] and Kohut's self psychology [14,15]. In a prior presentation [16], I introduced interspecies object relations theory (iORT). iORT builds on Balint's primary love [17,18] — the innate and dual object relation between an infant and its mother —, on the one hand, and on Panksepp's insight that from a neuroscientific perspective mammals share a set of innate basic emotions [6], on the other. In addition, evidence that emotions have interspecies potential delivers the basis for regarding human-animal relationships as a legitimate component of ORT and, hence, of Balint work.

This paper is structured as follows. The first section sketches my interpretation of human-animal relationships that is based on understanding Panksepp's basic emotions CARE and PLAY as primary object-love and primary object-empathy, respectively. The second section presents three cases of pet-owning patients that were presented during Balint work in which I participated as a group member. The third section closes the paper.

## 1. An interspecies object relations theory of human-animal relationships

The close bond between humans and their pets is the result of their daily interactions: hanging out and playing together, sharing space and food, and simply viewing one another as a family or pack member. But what exactly makes humans and animals interact in such a natural way? My answer is that this is due to interspecies empathy and care, two emotion-driven relations that can each be interpreted as a primary object relation. In contrast to a Freudian drive, a primary object relation is directed towards an object that is essential for mental development [17]. I argue that for a child's mental development not only are caretakers mentally formative and therefore non-arbitrary, but so are peers and pets.

I start out from Panksepp's neurobiological insight that animals and humans share a common set of primary-process emotions, each of them rooted in a subneocortical brain system [6]. We can think of his primary-process emotions as building blocks of mental development, in humans as well as in animals [19,20,21]. Particularly, I propose that Panksepp's CARE is pretty much what Balint's primary object-love stands for, i.e. the innate and unconditional caring and care-receiving relation between a mother and her infant [17,18]. What is important here is that "[t]his primitive-egoistic-form of love works according to the principle: what is good for me is right for you …; it assumes … that the partner's desires are identical with one's own [17:100]." Primary love is an "archaic, egotistic way of loving" [18:113]: the interests of the love-object do not matter, which does not mean that they are consciously neglected.

The next step is then to say that primary emotions are not necessarily directed to an object of one's own species. Thinking again of CARE/primary love, there are countless examples, including in the wild, of mother animals taking care of orphans of another species and raising them like their own offspring. Cross-species maternal care then delivers evidence of a first neurobiological basis for defining iORT.

Existing ORTs only regard a care giver — usually the mother — as an infant's primary object and the care relation between them as the only primary object relation. Even more, according to Balint "all later object-relations can be traced back to [primary object-love] [17:101]." I am not convinced that independent evidence exists for his view. If we just think of twins, obviously one twin is a non-arbitrary object for the other twin, which comes down to saying that peers are a substantial part of a subject's earliest mental development. Intuitively, what comes to mind first as primary interactions between twins and other peers growing up together, is touching, huddling, playing. This brings us to Panksepp's primary-process emotion PLAY, which — like CARE — I regard as a building block of mental development.

Mentally, PLAY can at best be traced back to what I call object-empathy, which captures the primary object relation between peers. Like primary love, primary empathy is egoistic in that it is about attributing one's own feelings to another object rather than attributing someone else's feelings to oneself, which is rather a sign of higher-order or learned empathy. Like primary love, I understand primary empathy as an archaic, self-oriented way of empathizing. The needs of the empathy-object do not matter, that is, they are not even recognized. Again, it is the principle of what-is-good-for-me-is-right-for-you that applies. Hence, I do not think of empathy as a developmental achievement but rather that it is biologically rooted in the neurophysiology of thermosensation. For example, if a pup in a litter feels cold, it will attribute this feeling to its littermates: they must feel cold as well. This attribution *is* primary empathy. Since each pup attributes this feeling to the other pups, the pups will huddle, warm each other and reach individual homeostasis through the group. Meeting this primary need as a group is less energetically costly than if each had to warm itself. I regard huddling as a very early form of playing: it creates socio-physical warmth between individuals. Saying that Panksepp's primary-order emotion PLAY has thermophysiological roots means that it is the neurobiological cradle of socio-emotional warmth. If a child wants to play with a group of peers, he or she is seeking socio-emotional warmth, a primary need. If they don't let him or her, the child will sense socio-emotional cold.

While in primary object-love there is neither equality nor parity between those providing care and those demanding it, primary empathy is directed towards objects of the same age, same group [22], same culture and, hence, with similar feelings: a subject can only empathize with his or her "missing twin" [23,16]. Exactly this sensation of some kind of equality is the major reason why according to Lewin twins and siblings are largely neglected in psychoanalysis: "the analyst's recognition of the central importance of the twin relationship and hence of the transference twin, would lead to an experience of the analyst feeling threatened with a loss of parental authority and power [24:5]." Therefore, it is psychoanalytic technique that stands in the way, not the phenomenon of object-empathy itself.

Independent studies show that animals are able to empathize with their fellow animals [25,26,27,28]. Further, evidence exists that animals can feel into humans [29,30]. The essence of the HAB is then affective coexistence, that is, being together for the sake of being together and yielding social warmth, both physically and emotionally. For example, a dog and a human playing with each other is one way of reaching this. Through their interaction dog and human become "peers" as they adapt their way of playing to each other's abilities. This kind of peer adaptation is also expected to happen when e.g. children of different ages play together: if the older ones do not adjust their way of playing to the younger ones, the resulting interaction may not be considered as play in its true sense.

In sum, interpreting Panksepp's CARE and PLAY as species-independent primary love and primary empathy, respectively, together with existing evidence that both object relations have interspecies potential provides the basis of iORT. This proposal along with other findings about the psychodynamic aspects of human-animal relationships [5,9-15] makes them a natural part of Balint work.

## 2. Animals in Balint cases

When a doctor reports on a relationship with a human patient in a Balint group, it is often mentioned — sometimes with more, sometimes fewer details — that this patient owns a pet. After such case presentations, when the group can ask for more information about the patient's family situation, questions regarding the pet are the exception. Similarly, pets are seldom part of free association during Balint work. In this section, I discuss three cases showing that this piece of seemingly irrelevant information can be quite revealing in various ways. This may convince those who are still skeptical to consider human-animal relationships as relevant to Balint work.

CASE 1 — *A family doctor A reports on a case of an elderly patient B who is suffering from increasing dementia. A has known B and most of B's family for a long time. It is becoming increasingly difficult for B's relatives to give B the care B needs at home. The family wants B to move into a residential home for people with dementia, but B doesn't want to as B's two dogs cannot move into this home. The relationship with the dogs is one of the few elements of B's life that has remained stable. Communication with the pets still works fine but B's interactions with people are noticeably decreasing. A is preparing for retirement and has handed the practice over to a younger colleague while A is still working there. It seems that the patient's family wants to hold on to A, which makes it difficult for A to hand over B to his colleague.*

Despite increasing dementia, the communication between the patient and the dogs appeared intact. I remember that during Balint work I was the only person who mentioned the dogs. I said that I was not surprised about them still being able to interact with each other. Since humans and their pets do so at the level of primary-process emotions, the patient's loss of cognitive abilities did not matter to the relationship with the dogs. By moving into a residential home, however, the patient would lose this source of socio-emotional warmth. Similarly, the presenter was preparing for retirement and made an age-related decision by selling the practice. Emotionally, however, it was still considered the presenter's practice. To me it seemed that the patient's conflict somehow mirrored the presenter's conflict and perhaps that was the reason why the case had been brought up.

CASE 2 — *A psychiatrist P reports on a 21-year-old anorexic patient Q, single, who started therapy on Q's mother's initiative. P cannot find access to Q and describes the relationship as superficial. P doesn't really know whether and how it could be deepened. Q's anorexia is currently under control. Q's mother is very present: not only did she organize the therapy for Q, she even represented Q once during a therapy session when Q was not feeling well that day. Q is a law student but is also thinking about starting a training as a horse farmer. Q has a horse, which is co-financed by Q's parents and cared for by the mother. The horse is housed in a performance-oriented riding stable, but Q is dissatisfied with it. The stable and paddock are perceived as too small, the amount of feed as too low. The animal needs more space. There is talk of selling the horse.*

Although the horse was a very central topic in the case presentation, at first it did not receive much attention during Balint work. I brought in that there is something very ambivalent about owning a horse. In human society, horses are seen as strong living beings, participating in competitions, kept in separate boxes, etc. In nature, horses are flight animals living in a herd. Hence, if kept appropriately, they need a lot of space, a lot of low-energy food spread over a long eating period and at least one other fellow horse. The patient felt that the horse was not kept appropriately. Did the patient feel not being kept appropriately either? The mother controlled both the patient and the horse. Both of them did not have a partner, both were being fed by her. The only solution for the horse the patient could think of was not to change the horse-unfriendly situation but to get rid of the animal by selling it. The only solution for the patient was to refuse the mother's food, which amounts to getting rid of oneself.

CASE 3 — *A family doctor F reports on an alcoholic patient G, around 60 years old, to whom F had sent the police after F could not reach G by telephone. F was very worried about G's health situation because G hadn't shown up at F's practice for a long time. G had developed severe heart failure as a result of the addiction. The police found out on site that G was not at home because G had been admitted to a clinic, apparently on G's own initiative. Even after the police intervention, G did not contact F, which F interpreted as meaning that G had resentments about the intervention. F now felt guilty for having initiated it. In the case report it was also mentioned that G lived alone and had two cats. F found G to be endearing.*

During Balint work on this case, the cats were mentioned by a group member ridiculing the patient who supposedly could only care for two cats. I objected that the bond the patient had with these cats was worth more than this group member could imagine. Not only did it show that the patient was able to care for other living beings, namely, for two cats — even though or perhaps because, like alcoholics, animals are considered low in social hierarchy. Cats are freedom-loving animals: they only come if they want to, they can only be petted as long as they want to. To me it felt that for the very same reason the patient did not contact the doctor. That is, I didn't intuit any resentment over the police intervention, but rather that the patient wanted to be free to decide whether or not to see the family doctor.

## 3. Concluding remarks

Integrating human-animal relationships into a framework that is compatible with ORT and addressing the presence of animals in Balint cases, I hope to have shown that when a Balint group is open-minded towards interspecies relationships, this is a gain of the group's output.

At this point two remarks need to be added. The first one is that this paper is not a call to humanize animals but rather to reflect that on a vegetative level of sensation humans and animals share a common denominator. This requires openness with respect to species-relevant characteristics of those animals many humans share their homes and lives with.

The second remark is about the effect of the ambivalent ways in which society values and deals with animals. On the one hand, animals are described as valuable for a variety of reasons: they perform well in sports, they have exceptional characteristics for a certain breed, they are always loyal to their owner, they produce good meat, etc. However, in the very same society the treatment of animals is often unworthy: there is indifference towards their fate, cost efficiency is a priority in their healthcare, they are generally perceived as inferior to humans, etc. Veterinarians are confronted with this ambivalence on a daily basis. Interestingly, when I presented veterinary cases during Balint work, often the very same ambivalence emerged in the groups working on these cases. Even though this mirror effect may contribute to the overall understanding of animal-related Balint cases, differentiating the sociological status of a human-animal relationship from its psychological interpretation is necessary if we want to arrive at the emotional level at which humans and animals meet.

## Acknowledgments

Past experience has taught me that it is not always a given that as a veterinarian you will be seen as a fully-fledged analytical mind and on an equal footing. Therefore, I am grateful to the Program Committee for this opportunity to present my work. I would also like to thank two anonymous reviewers for their valuable comments on an earlier version of this paper. For her inspiring support while I was creating the final version, my special thanks go to E.K. Knowlton. All remaining errors are my own.

## References

[1] Goldberg K (2018) Considerations in counseling veterinarians: addressing suffering in those who care for animals. In: Kogan L, Blazina C (eds.) Clinician's guide to treating companion animal issues: addressing human-animal interaction. Amsterdam, Elsevier: 241-434.
[2] Van Geenhoven V (2020) Balintgruppenarbeit für Tiermediziner: die Aufarbeitung beruflicher Interaktionen als Qualitätssicherung und Burnout-Prophylaxe [Balint group work for veterinarians: catching up on professional interactions as quality assurance and burnout prophylaxis]. Deutsches Tierärzteblatt 68: 315-318.
[3] Van Geenhoven V (2021) Über professionelle Beziehungen zu Heimtieren und ihren Besitzern: die tiermedizinische Triade und ihre Folgen für die Balintarbeit [About professional relationships with pets and their owners: the veterinary triad and its implications for Balint work]. Balint-Journal 22: 109-119.
[4] Serpell JA, Paul ES (2011) Pets in the family: an evolutionary perspective. In Shackelford TK, Salmon CA (eds.) The Oxford handbook of evolutionary family psychology. New York, Oxford University Press: 298-310.
[5] Roth B (2005) Pets and psychoanalysis: a clinical contribution. Psychoanal Rev 92: 453-467.
[6] Panksepp J (1998) Affective neuroscience: the foundations of human and animal emotions. New York, Oxford University Press.
[7] Amiot CE, Bastian B (2015). Toward a psychology of human-animal relations. Psychol Bull 141: 6-47.
[8] Hosey G, Melfi V (2014) Human-animal interactions, relationships and bonds: a review and analysis of the literature. Int J Comp Psychol 27: 117-142.
[9] Meggeson S (2021) A dog in the room: interspecies intersubjectivity in relational psychotherapy. In: Silbert J, Frasca J (eds.) Animals as the third in relational psychotherapy: exploring theory, frame and practice. New York, Routledge: 48-54.

[10] Crawford KE, Worsham NL, Swinehart ER (2006) Benefits derived from companion animals, and the use of the term "attachment". Anthrozoös 19: 98-112.

[11] Field NP, Orsini L, Gavish R, Packman W (2009) Role of attachment in response to pet loss. Death Stud 33: 334-355.

[12] Kurdek LA (2008) Pet dogs as attachment figures. J Soc Pers Rel 25: 247-266.

[13] Blazina C (2011) Life after loss: psychodynamic perspectives on a continuing bonds approach with "pet companion". In: Blazina C, Boyraz G, Shen-Miller D (eds.) The psychology of the human-animal bond. New York, Springer: 203-224.

[14] Brown S-E (2007) Companion animals as selfobjects. Anthrozoös 20: 329-343.

[15] Rachmani V (2021) Relational creatures: the selfobject functions of dogs in psychoanalytic theory and practice. In: Silbert J, Frasca J (eds.) Animals as the third in relational psychotherapy: exploring theory, frame and practice. New York, Routledge: 26-48.

[16] Van Geenhoven V (2023) Pets, primary empathy and the missing twin: a Balintian interpretation of PLAY, CARE and emotional contagion in human-animal interactions. Poster, 22nd Annual Meeting of the International Neuropsychoanalysis Society (NPSA), Tel Aviv.

[17] Balint M (1937) Early developmental states of the ego: primary object love. In: Balint M (1952) Primary love and psychoanalytic technique. London, Hogarth Press Ltd: 89-108.

[18] Balint A (1939) Love for the mother and mother-love. In: Balint M (1952) Primary love and psychoanalytic technique. London, Hogarth Press Ltd: 108-127.

[19] Panksepp J (2012) How primary-process emotional systems guide child development: ancestral regulators of human happiness, thriving, and suffering. In: Narvaez D, Panksepp J, Schore AN, Gleason TR (eds.) Evolution, early experience and human development: from research to practice and policy. New York, Oxford University Press: 74-94.

[20] Panksepp J (2017) Affective consciousness. In: Schneider S, Velmans M (eds.) The Blackwell companion to consciousness. Oxford, Wiley: 141-156.

[21] Turnbull OH, Bar A (2020) Animal minds: the case for emotion, based on neuroscience. Neuropsychoanalysis 22: 109-128.

[22] Miyazono K, Inarimori K (2021) Empathy, altruism, and group identification. Front Psychol 12: 749315.

[23] Burlingham DT (1946) The fantasy of having a twin. Psychoanal Study Child 1: 205-210.

[24] Lewin V (2014) The twin in the transference, 2nd edition. New York, Routledge.

[25] de Waal FBM (2007) Do animals *feel* empathy? Sci Am Mind 18(6): 28-35.

[26] Panksepp J, Panksepp JB (2013) Toward a cross-species understanding of empathy. Trends Neurosci 36: 489-496.

[27] Ferretti V, Papaleo F (2019) Understanding others: emotion recognition in humans and other animals. Genes Brain Behav 18: e12544.

[28] Kim S-W, Kim M, Shin H-S (2021) Affective empathy and prosocial behavior in rodents Curr Opin Neurobiol 68: 181-189.

[29] Katayama M, Kubo T, Yamakawa T, Fujiwara K, Nomoto K, Ikeda K, Mogi K, Nagasawa M, Kikusui T (2019) Emotional contagion from humans to dogs is facilitated by duration of ownership. Front Psychol 10: 1678.

[30] Van Bourg J, Patterson JE, Wynne CDL (2020) Pet dogs *(Canis lupus familiaris)* release their trapped and distressed owners: individual variation and evidence of emotional contagion. PLoS One 15: e0231742.

# Chapter 4

# Cultivating Understanding and Compassion through Balint

Eddo De Lang, MD
Family Physician (retired)
Mary Washington Family Medicine Residency Program
Fredericksburg, VA, USA
Wright Center for Graduate Medical Education
National Family Medicine Residency
Washington, DC, USA
eddo.delang@gmail.com

## Abstract

A story about my journey through forty plus years of practicing Family Medicine and the importance of building relationships with patients. The story describes how building those relationships has enriched my experience of practicing primary care medicine. Ultimately this led me to rediscover Balint after many years practicing without it. Becoming a Balint Co-Leader in Residency Programs has been a very positive experience for me by letting Residents experience early in their careers that relationship building with patients and sharing dilemmas in a Balint Group can lead to enhanced satisfaction in their career. Working in an otherwise fairly hostile environment in today's "Health Care Industry" can be positively compensated by regularly practicing reflective techniques such as Balint.

When I decided after four decades of practicing Family Medicine that it was time to focus on some other interests in life, reflection became a more prominent component of my thoughts. After so many years pondering about difficult situations that so many of "my" patients faced I became more and more aware that it left me wondering about my role as a physician and how that had affected my being. From an early age on I had decided that practicing medicine would be what I wanted to do. My role model was a Family Physician in the small town in the Netherlands where I grew up. I could see myself in his role. Being able to help people overcome diseases seemed like an excellent career choice. That choice has not disappointed me. The journey in medical school at the University of Groningen in the Netherlands made me more and more curious about the structure and functioning of the human body. Learning the basic principles of psychology and psychiatry helped me understand how the mind plays an essential role in the experience of it all. What medical school could not teach me was how working with this knowledge and creating relationships with patients would change me even more over time.

The experiential learning curve of life in medicine is much less steep than the didactic learning curve in medical school and thereafter, but the former has created more profound and lasting effects for me. Looking back, reminiscing and reflecting on situations that I have encountered, the one theme that prevails is the richness of having been able to create meaningful relationships with patients. Sharing the good and bad with patients gave me purpose. It often felt that my profession was a hybrid of being a physician, a social worker and hopefully a companion for the patients who crossed my path in life. Sometimes it even felt like taking confession when I encountered someone in great psychological peril or need. It gave my professional life depth in a way that would have been difficult to match by having done something else.

I remember that many years ago I was called to the Emergency Department to admit one of my patients. Several weeks before that call I had a difficult visit with the couple in our office. Initially I felt some hostility during that visit. When I told them that I felt some negative vibes in the room it became clear that they were afraid. He had several serious chronic medical problems and they expected a poor outcome. That fear was justified and we had a long conversation about prognosis, expectations and personal preferences. Their main concern was that they questioned if I would be available in times of need, they needed someone who knew they could count on, but they did not expect miracles. They did not want to get lost in the hospital cared for by an unknown hospitalist, who would just treat his illness, but had no eye for him as a person. Little did I know then that only a few weeks later he would end up in the ER and die while in the process of being admitted by me. I believe that if I had not had that conversation in the office a few weeks prior it would have created a very difficult situation for his wife and myself. When he died she only wanted emotional support, she understood that it had been an expectation and she was accepting of the poor outcome. Afterward she continued to be my patient for many years and that shared experience had truly deepened our relationship and helped us both to move forward in life.

What we learned in medical school was to maintain a certain emotional distance to the patient to retain medical objectivity. Getting emotionally involved in that relationship would somehow cloud our judgements, but is that actually true? I have found that it is virtually impossible to avoid creating a true relationship with the patient. Good or bad, it is part of human interactions, unless we attempt to dehumanize our clinical tasks. Our medical environment has done a formidable job at succeeding in minimizing the importance of relationship building: by following protocols, using electronic medical records and dealing with impersonal administrative systems in the healthcare industry. Renaming medical arts into "Health Care Industry" is probably very telling in where we have arrived. Maybe it is time to put relationship building back into the frontline of our work and coupled with our clinical tasks we can be trusted to do the best job we are trained for. We can push the rest into the least important back room or perhaps even the room everyone forgot was there. Maybe someone else can take over the administrative and documentation tasks instead?

During most of my working years I did not have access to Balint Groups, although I had been exposed to it during my first Family Medicine Residency in the Netherlands in the late 70's to 1980. A family physician in the group practice where I had my first outpatient Family Medicine Residency rotations was an active Balint Group member and told me passionately about how it helped him deal with difficult patient relationships. I was curious, but could not join him in the group, because I would have been a temporary member. During our weekly didactic sessions back at the Medical School in Groningen we had Balint-like experiences where we shared difficult clinician-patient relationship issues and speculated about what could be happening, but the resident group did not actually "take the case" from the presenter. After I had moved to the US in 1987, I had to redo my Residency. I was surprised that in the Miami Residency we entirely focused on clinical training without reflective exercises. That made me believe that Balint was not part of the US medical community and I never explored it further until about 2016. Practicing for many years in a small rural town in the US, it was at times challenging to find a way to process difficult relationships. There was no safe place to share my dilemmas in the small community. There were no accessible existing Balint Groups as far as I knew. When I changed from working in our private practice to becoming a Rural Family Medicine Residency Program Director toward the end of my career I was looking for a different, non-clinical method to try to deepen the experience of practicing medicine for our residents. I wanted to take them away from just clinical thinking and help them experience what had touched me most: creating a long-term relationship with many patients. I finally discovered that Balint did also exist in the US and decided to attend my first Leadership Intensive in 2018. That experience helped me to see that introducing Balint as part of medical training could be very helpful.

Working with residents I had discovered that their emphasis was mainly on learning practical skills, solving case management questions and finding answers to medical problems. For me the patient-clinician relationships had evolved to be the most important, something I wanted the young colleagues to experience as well. I thought that Balint could be a good method to emphasize the importance of building strong relationships with patients. Showing an effort to build these meaningful relationships for me is a sign of respect for those we attempt to treat, for our profession and for ourselves. Reducing our profession as clinicians to a problem solving and management concept does very little for us as fellow human beings of those we want to help. We cannot see our patients like cars in the repair shop where the technician plugs the car into a computer and let the machine tell us what is wrong. Becoming our patient's partner in finding ways to reduce suffering opens the door to a deeper level of understanding of each other. Finding that more gratifying relationship experience touches on the reasons why I think I wanted to become that small community physician. It has helped me to avoid burn-out, a disease so easily acquired in today's emphasis on promoting efficiency and productivity.

Starting and continuing to lead a Balint group has been one of the most gratifying experiences since I decided to retire from gainful employment several years ago. I look forward to leading each group and it continues to challenge my mind by staying focused on the presentation, nudging the group to look in areas where they can discover what was not yet considered and enjoying the palpable outcomes of the group's discovery tour. It has also helped me to look beyond the obvious, be truly curious about what drives the other human being and why I feel excited when I can still meet that person in need by practicing my profession in my volunteer job. Looking the patient in the eyes and seeing a reflection of recognition when I attempt to show true interest in that person is something that can never be achieved by artificial intelligence. Making the correct diagnosis and starting a treatment plan in our work is only where our task begins, not where it should end.

In a world that is so full of conflict, controversy and uncertainty I have found that residents have a growing need to learn how to speculate about relationships with the patients they treat. Speculation does not appear to be an intuitive activity for many, but an acquired gift that can be developed. The slow transformation from looking for answers to appreciating the freedom of thought in careful speculation is wonderful to witness. The added dimensions and the richness of empathy of the group transmitted to the clinician and the patient makes me think about how helpful it would be if our world leaders would Balint their relationships and speculate about what the other side may be experiencing. At the moment we perhaps can only do that in our Balint Groups here and at home. But we can attempt being an example of what could take place in other areas on our planet.

Let's continue focusing on the wellbeing of our patients with the aid of processing our dilemmas together through Balint while keeping ourselves healthy as well.

# Balint Groups and Health Professionals' Perceived Well-Being – An Israeli Study

Ruth Kannai, MD
Clalit Health Services and Ben-Gurion University of the Negev, Faculty
of Health Sciences, Department of Family Medicine
Beer Sheva, Israel
rkannai@gmail.com

Aya Biderman, MD
Clalit Health Services and Ben-Gurion University of the Negev, Faculty
of Health Sciences, Department of Family Medicine
Beer Sheva, Israel
abid@bgu.ac.il

Tamar Freud, PhD
Clalit Health Services and Ben-Gurion University of the Negev, Faculty
of Health Sciences, Dept. of Family Medicine
Beer Sheva, Israel
freudt@bgu.ac.il

Shai Krontal, MD
Department of Family Medicine, Maccabi Healthcare Services
Department of Family Medicine, Faculty of Medicine
Tel Aviv University
Tel Aviv, Israel
krontal@gmail.com

## Abstract

Health professionals' well-being is a goal that impacts patients' care, their satisfaction and outcomes. Previous studies that have demonstrated the positive effects of Balint Groups (BGs) are descriptive and based on small sample sizes. We evaluated the perceptions of health professionals who participated in BGs, to identify the factors related to their perceived well-being.

In January and February 2023, we performed a cross-sectional study. We distributed a questionnaire to members of the Israeli internet network of Family physicians, to a mailing list of the Israeli BG association and during a conference for Family Medicine teachers. The questionnaire included demographic and professional information and a 5-point Likert scale for the level of agreement with a list of 15 statements regarding BGs. We received 142 responses, most of whom were family physicians. More than half were teachers and/or leaders in the medical system.

Respondents who had participated in BGs reported a reduction in burnout, increased empathy, enhanced professional identity and better relationships with patients and colleagues. Those who attended BGs for more than 5 years reported significantly more positive outcomes compared to those who attended less than 1 year. In a logistic regression analysis, we found two factors significantly associated with self-reported well-being: attending BGs for more than five years and perceiving BGs as a means for relieving burnout. Participation in BGs seems to have a positive impact on healthcare professionals' perceived well-being and professional development. The findings suggest that medical organizations should encourage the regular availability of BGs to support health professionals' well-being.

*****

Health care professionals' (HCPs) burnout has been linked to decreased productivity, harm to patients and a decline in the quality of treatment (1). Whereas health professionals' well-being is a goal that impacts patients' care, their satisfaction and outcomes. Several studies described the positive effects of Balint Groups on increasing job satisfaction and preventing burnout (2-4).

In this study, we aimed to assess the perception of a large group of health professionals who participated in BGs, regarding its impact on their perceived personal and professional well-being, and to learn what factors are related to these positive outcomes.

This cross-sectional study was performed during 1-2/2023. We distributed questionnaires through the Israeli internet network of Family doctors, the mailing list of the Israeli Balint Association and participants of the Himar (Israeli Society of Family Medicine Teachers) conference. The questionnaire included the demographic and professional background of respondents and a 5-point Likert scale regarding their agreement with 15 positive and negative statements, regarding their experiences with BGs.

The mean age of respondents was 51.07 ($\pm$10.3), 103 females (75.2%), 113 (81.3%) born in Israel. Most respondents were board certified family physicians (84.8%), who completed their academic studies in Israel. About half of the respondents had a professional experience of more than 20 years. An impressive number of the participants (82.7%) were involved in teaching, and over 50% were engaged in management positions (50.4%).

Concerning their experience with Balint Groups, 38.0% were actively involved in a BG, while 47.2% have participated in the past and 14.8% have never joined a BG. Among those who participated, 32.5% did so for less than a year, 32.5% for 1-4 years, 17.9% for 5-9 years, and 17.1% for more than 10 years. More than 20 % of the respondents currently lead a BG.

Participants rated their agreement with several statements concerning involvement in their most recent Balint Group. (fig. 1) More than half of the BG participants (56.7%) answered that their involvement in BG is important/very important, for their professional well-being, while 22.5% responded that it was not important or not important at all.

Among 21 respondents who never participated in a BG, the main reasons for non-participation were organizational: it was offered at the expense of private or family time or that there was no BG in their area of residence, or that it was not accessible to them. Only two respondents did not believe in the usefulness of the group, and one did not trust the group.

In all positive statements there was a significant difference in their score, in relation to the duration of participation. These differences were markedly significant between less than a year of participation in the BG and 5 years or more. Regarding the importance of participation in a BG for their professional well-being, participants of more than 5 years scored significantly better than those who participated in the BG for less than a year.

Participants with less than a year of experience were more likely to report feeling uncomfortable sharing their cases, while those who had been in the group for a longer period, particularly for more than five years, were more comfortable sharing.

In a logistic regression analysis (table 1), we found only two factors significantly associated with perceived well-being: attending BGs for more than five years (OR=7.158, 95% CI 1.65-31.058) and perceiving BGs as a means of relieving burnout (OR=3.074, 95% CI 1.508-6.269). Other factors, including age, gender, professional experience, and involvement in teaching or management, were not related to perceived well-being.

The results of this study provide evidence for the positive effects of BG participation on healthcare professionals' well-being and professional development. These findings are consistent with previous research indicating that BG participation can reduce burnout, increase empathy and communication skills, and enhance professional identity and relationships with patients and colleagues. We found that the longer the duration of participation in BGs, the more positive outcomes, especially for those who attended BGs for more than five years.

This finding might be seen as a combination of "cause" and "effect": not only that the BG has a positive impact on the attendants, but also that those who experience these positive effects continue to attend BGs for longer periods of time. A similar connection can exist between the increase in wellbeing and the perceived reduction in burnout.

The study also highlights some of the barriers to participation in BG, such as conflicts with private or family time and lack of availability in certain geographical areas. There could be other hidden reasons for avoiding joining BGs, such as difficulty in sharing one's feelings, and in disclosing vulnerabilities with colleagues. Addressing these barriers may be important for increasing participation rates and extending the benefits of BGs to more healthcare professionals.

Based on these findings, we emphasize that establishing BGs should be the responsibility of employers, such as the Health Ministry, HMO's, hospitals, and professional unions. The Balint Association in Israel is currently working towards establishing more groups in hospital departments and in large clinics for selected professional groups or for multi professional teams.

In our study, there were fewer respondents from minority or immigrant backgrounds, lower than their proportion in the population. This may be related to different cultural or educational backgrounds, where it is less acceptable to share or even to express one's feelings and difficulties among colleagues.

It is crucial that healthcare workers prioritize compassion, not just for their patients but also for themselves. Engaging in Balint groups offers a space for self-compassion, allowing participants to step away from the competitive environment and explore the vulnerabilities inherent in doctor-patient relationships. Embracing self-compassion is essential for cultivating the well-being and resilience of those in the demanding fields of healthcare.

The study relied on self-report measures, which may be subject to biases and inaccuracies, such as "social desirability bias". Future research could incorporate more objective measures of outcomes such as patient satisfaction or clinical outcomes. We believe that it is the ethical responsibility of employers, to ensure the professional well-being of their employees. Healthcare organizations may benefit from considering BGs as part of a comprehensive approach for preventing and addressing burnout and promoting a culture of reflective practice and professional growth.

To launch and maintain such a program, it is essential to have visionaries who can lead the effort. Achieving this important goal requires collaboration from all professionals involved. As the saying goes, 'It takes a village' (6).

## References

1. Hull SK, DiLalla LF, Dorsey JK. Prevalence of health-related behaviors among physicians and medical trainees. Acad Psychiatry. 2008;32(1):31-38. doi: 10.1176/appi.ap.32.1.31. PMID: 18270278.

2. Shorer Y, Rabin S, Zlotnik M, Cohen N, Nadav M, Shiber A. [Balint Group as a means for burnout prevention and improvement of therapist-patient relationship in a general hospital – The Soroka experience] Harefuah. 2016;155(2):115-118, 130. Hebrew. PMID: 27215125.

3. Stojanovic-Tasic M, Latas M, Milosevic N, et al (2018) Is Balint training associated with the reduced burnout among primary health care doctors? Libyan Journal of Medicine. 13:1. DOI: 10.1080/19932820.2018.1440123

4. Kjeldmand D, Holmström I. Balint groups as a means to increase job satisfaction and prevent burnout among general practitioners. Ann Fam Med. 2008;6(2):138-145. doi: 10.1370/afm.813. PMID: 18332406; PMCID: PMC2267420.

5. Huang L, Harsh J, Cui H, et al. A Randomized Controlled Trial of Balint Groups to Prevent Burnout Among Residents in China. Front Psychiatry. 2020;10:957. doi: 10.3389/fpsyt.2019.00957. PMID: 32116808; PMCID: PMC7026367.

6. Krontal S. Balint Infrastructure in a Large Tertiary Hospital in Israel. Balint International conference, Porto, Portugal 2019. https://www.balintinternational.com/wp-content/uploads/2019/11/Proceedings-book-Porto-2019.pdf

**Figure 1 – Level of agreement with the statements concerning participation in the most recent BG\* (N=121)**

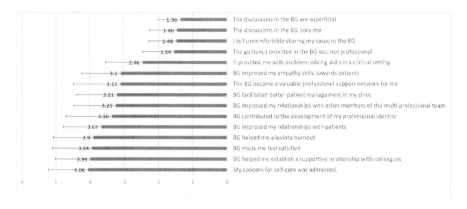

Scale of 1-5: 1 indicates complete disagreement and 5 indicates substantial agreement.
BG: Balint Group

**Table 1: Logistic regression analysis to determine factors related to self-perception of professional well-being.**

| Variable | OR | P value | 95%CI |
|---|---|---|---|
| Age | 0.996 | 0.909 | 0.933-1.063 |
| Gender | 2.29 | 0.177 | 0.689-7.613 |
| Management position | 0.577 | 0.279 | 0.213-1.561 |
| Teaching | 3.56 | 0.08 | 0.859-14.752 |
| Seniority in the profession | 0.516 | 0.337 | 0.133-1.994 |
| | | | |
| Length of participation in BGs: | | | |
| Less than a year | Reference | | |
| 1-4 years | 3.329 | 0.058 | 0.962-11.516 |
| 5+ years | 7.158 | **0.009** | 1.65-31.058 |
| BG improved my relationships with patients | 1.043 | 0.897 | 0.55-1.977 |
| BG helped me alleviate burnout | 3.074 | **0.002** | 1.508-6.269 |

# A Survey of Knowledge, Skills, and Attitudes Gained by Medical Students Participating in Balint Groups

Tamatha Psenka, MD
Medical University of South Carolina, Department of Family Medicine,
Charleston, South Carolina, USA
psenkatm@musc.edu

Clive Brock, MD
Medical University of South Carolina, Dept, of Family Medicine (retired)
Charleston, South Carolina, USA
clive.d.brock@gmail.com

Frank Dornfest, MD
Oregon Health and Science University, Department of Family Medicine
(retired) Loveland, Colorado, USA
frankdornfest@gmail.com

Alan Johnston, PhD
Medical University of South Carolina, Department of Family Medicine,
Charleston, South Carolina, USA
johnsonah39@gmail.com

Laurel Milberg, PhD
University of Pittsburgh School of Medicine, Dept. of Family Medicine
(retired)
Pittsburgh, Pennsylvania, USA
laurelmilberg@gmail.com

Paul Scott, MD
University of Pittsburgh School of Medicine, Dept. of Family Medicine
(retired)
Pittsburgh, Pennsylvania, USA

paulcp1@gmail.com

# Abstract

Balint groups have been used in graduate medical education resulting in improved doctor-patient interaction skills. Unfortunately, only a handful of American medical schools offer a Balint group experience to their students, leaving a curriculum mainly devoid of this effective way of teaching about and developing such skills.

A survey measuring key knowledge, attitudes, and skills acquired through Balint training was developed by the History and Continuity Committee of the American Balint Society and distributed in late 2023 to lists of known national and international leaders of medical student Balint groups. This work in progress will present and assess survey responses and outline next steps. By identifying specific knowledge, attitudes, and skills gained by participants in current medical student Balint groups, the hope is to better inform medical schools and their accrediting bodies on the timing, planning, and anticipated outcomes of this training, thereby encouraging its inclusion in medical school training.

**Rationale:** "The Flexner Report of 1910 transformed the nature and process of medical education in America with a resulting elimination of proprietary schools and the establishment of the biomedical model as the gold standard of medical training. This transformation occurred in the aftermath of the report, which embraced scientific knowledge and advancement as the defining ethos of the modern physician. American medicine profited immeasurably from the scientific advances that this system allowed but ... created an ....excellence in science that was not balanced by a comparable excellence in clinical caring." (1)

As a result, medical education has often failed to train physicians in the art of communication and the skillful use of the doctor patient relationship as a therapeutic tool, which would significantly enhance the disclosure of factors and feelings immediately relevant in the encounter. Poor communication in healthcare can contribute to inaccurate diagnoses, unnecessary laboratory work or consultations, poor medical adherence, perpetuation of health inequities, and dissatisfaction on the part of both patient and clinician.

Balint group training was developed by psychoanalyst Michael and clinical social worker Enid Balint in the 1950s, after World War II, to provide a group learning environment and support for general practitioners to improve their understanding and skill in management of internal and external factors which were impacting themselves and their role in the patient-doctor relationship. Since that time, the use of the Balint method in graduate medical education has been shown to improve self-awareness and communication skills, appreciation of the importance of the doctor-patient relationship, increase in empathy for the patient, decrease in burnout, and improvement in self-management around difficult emotional aspects of the encounter. (2-4)

Balint group training creates a safe, group learning environment in which students can begin to understand themselves in relation to a patient and vice versa. This method encourages consideration of both internal and external factors which may be influencing the relationship. It facilitates both individual and group learning regarding intentional exploration of differing perspectives. Qualitative analyses of Balint groups for medical students have identified common themes of: more awareness of personal thoughts and feelings related to patients, increased awareness of different perspectives of peers, more awareness and tolerance for uncertainty, a safe environment to enable vulnerability, forming professional identity within the medical hierarchy. (3,4)

Unfortunately, only a handful of American medical schools offer a Balint group experience to their students, leaving a curriculum often devoid of this effective way of teaching about and developing doctor patient relationship skills. This presentation outlines steps taken to lay the groundwork for Balint groups' widespread introduction into undergraduate medical education, surprisingly, a "new" setting for Balint training.

**Method**: The History and Continuity Committee (HCC) of the American Balint Society (ABS) took on the goal of eventually introducing relationship skills as core competencies into the requirements for medical school education, seeking acceptance for this requirement from the Liaison Committee on Medical Education (LCGME) an accrediting body for educational programs at schools of medicine in the US and Canada, using a two-pronged approach.

1) Seasoned ABS Balint group leaders conducted four session Balint groups comprised of medical students from all over the US, an extra-curricular, voluntary activity meant to spark student interest in having Balint groups as part of their medical education.

2) By identifying specific knowledge, attitudes, and skills gained by participants in current Balint groups for medical students, the hope is to better inform medical schools and their accrediting bodies on the timing, planning, and anticipated outcomes of this training.

A survey measuring key knowledge, attitudes, and skills acquired through Balint training was developed by the HCC of the ABS through an iterative process of identifying from literature and experience what could be learned through participation in a Balint group. This IRB approved instrument (see Table 1) was distributed in late 2023 to lists of known national and international leaders of medical student Balint groups. These lists were obtained through the ABS and the International Balint Federation (IBF). The survey was distributed anonymously through REDcaps. Recipients were contacted by email on 3 separate occasions over a 60-day period for completion.

**Results**: This work in progress will present and assess survey responses and outline next steps.

### References
1. Duffy, T. The Flexner Report---100 Years Later. Yale J. of Bio/Med, 2011. Sept: 84(3) 269-276.

2. Yazdankhahfard M, Haghani F, Omid A. The Balint group and its application in medical education: A systematic review. J Educ Health Promot. 2019 Jun 27;8:124. doi: 10.4103/jehp.jehp_423_18. PMID: 31334276; PMCID: PMC6615135.

3. Player M, Freedy JR, Diaz V, Brock C, Chessman A, Thiedke C, Johnson A. The role of Balint group training in the professional and personal development of family medicine residents. Int J Psychiatry Med. 2018 Jan-Mar;53(1-2):24-38. doi: 10.1177/0091217417745289. Epub 2017 Dec 13. PMID: 29235909.

4. Ng et al. Modelling vulnerability: qualitative study of the Balint process for medical students. BMC Med Educ (2022)22:436. https://doi.org/10.1186/s12909-022-03508-2

5. Torppa, MA et al. A qualitative analysis of student Balint groups in medical education: Contexts and triggers of case presentations and discussion themes. Patient Educ and Counseling 72 (2008) 5-11.

**Table 1. Survey for Leaders of Balint Groups for Medical Students**

**Questions: As a result of participating in a Balint group, medical students**

Can identify the centrality of clinician-patient relationship in medical care.

Demonstrate curiosity about each patient as a unique person within their social context.

Better understand nonverbalized patient needs.

Show increased understanding of the patient's concern over their own drive to be competent and "fix things."

Can acknowledge realistic limitations of the clinician's role.

Have better appreciation of the diversity of perspective and experience of patients.

Have better appreciation of the diversity of perspective and experience of peers.

Develop empathy skills through case-based group experiential learning.

Can use self-reflection and awareness of self and other to inform diagnostic accuracy.

Improve active listening skills.

Increase self-awareness of their emotional reactions and how this impacts their care of patients.

Are more skillful in their use of self in a therapeutic relationship.

Increase awareness of their own implicit biases

Increase their ability to self-manage discomfort and uncertainty arising from patient encounter.

Increase their situational awareness of moments which may trigger lapses in professional behavior.

Survey participants were asked to rate the questions on a scale from 1 to 5:
1 = Strongly Disagree, 2 = Disagree, 3 = Neutral, 4 = Agree, 5 = Strongly Agree. N/A = cannot rate.

# Balint in the Wilderness

Sandra Relyea, PA-C
Peninsula Children's Clinic
Port Angeles, Washington, USA
sandrajr8@gmail.com

Francis Chu, MD
Residency Program Director, Kaiser Permanente
San Jose, California, USA
francis.n.chu@kp.org

Geoffrey Margo, MD
Private Practice, Psychiatry
Philadelphia, Pennsylvania, USA
gmargo@me.com

Katherine Margo, MD
Department of Family Medicine and Community Health
Perelman School of Medicine at University of Pennsylvania
Philadelphia, Pennsylvania, USA
katiemargo@gmail.com

## Abstract

The American Balint Society sponsored a 6-day, 5-night river rafting event, which included 10 Balint sessions over 6 days, in June of 2023. The event included 22 participants, including 4 credentialed Balint Leaders, 15 Balint Group members/participants, and 3 guests of individual Balint participants. Ten continuing medical education credits were awarded to Balint participants at the end of the event. One overall intent of the event was to explore the viability of the juxtaposition of a wilderness experience with traditional Balint Group sessions. Event coordinators were especially interested in what effects this unprecedented setting would have on the function and effectiveness of Balint participation on group members as well as what unique challenges it might present for group leaders.

## Introduction

This event initially came about because of two passions of one of the authors (SR), Balint and wilderness. She thought that the combination of these two passions would work well for a number of reasons, including testing out the viability of Balint work in a very different setting, unfamiliar and challenging for many participants, but also free of the distractions of work and

technology - no signal in the wilderness! It was hoped also that the combination of wilderness

and Balint work might appeal to a younger demographic and people who do their clinical work

outside of an academic institution. In order to realize this vision, 3 additional credentialed leaders, who were equally taken by this new juxtaposition, were recruited. As faculty for this adventure, we asked ourselves what effect this unique setting would have on participants' feelings of safety, focus and mental containment in a Balint group. How would exposure to rain, wind, cold, sun and a degree of physical risk affect group function and cohesion? There is nowhere to escape or retreat to in the middle of an outdoor wilderness devoid of roads, trails, durable housing, and communication with the rest of the world. We concluded that it was an exciting project to pilot.

## Discussion

The trip:

The wilderness experience was built around a six-day, five-night rafting journey down the Salmon River from Corn Creek to Carey Creek, Idaho, a distance of just over 80 miles of class III+ to IV wild and scenic whitewater in the middle of the Idaho Rocky Mountains.

Arrangements were made with Momentum River Expeditions, a professional rafting company, to guide us down the river. They were happy to work with us to incorporate Balint group sessions

as part of the daily routine on the trip. June was chosen for the event as the river would be high with spring snow melt, allowing us to move down river quickly, which in turn provided time

for two Balint groups a day, one after breakfast, and one before dinner. Momentum made all the

logistical arrangements and we were in their hands once we arrived in Boise. They provided

transportation to and from the river, the rafts, tents, sleeping bags, food (delicious! with wine pairings) and other needed equipment.

Through the American Balint Society (ABS) Events Committee, ABS approval of the event was obtained. A call was put out through the ABS and the International Balint Federation (IBF) inviting participation. Within two weeks there were enough registrants to confirm the trip.

During the months prior to launch, many questions were fielded from registrants regarding what physical abilities (generally good health), prior experience (none), clothing (layered), flying (in tiny planes over mountainous terrain), etc. would be required or expected.

A hearty crew arrived in Boise to be flown in small aircraft across the Sawtooth Mountains to our launch site. There were some minor glitches along the way. Our start on the river was delayed by a few hours because one of the small airplanes assigned to fly us over the mountains had a dead battery, so one plane had to make two trips. One participant fell out of her raft once but was quickly brought back in and found it an inspiring experience! Otherwise, the trip was almost seamless, and we have nothing but praise for the people who guided us.

Along the way we learned to paddle a raft in whitewater, visited homestead and other historic sites, viewed First Nations pictographs, and soaked in a hot spring. One of the raft guides had been down the Salmon more than 40 times over the years and he was a wellspring of information about the river, its history, and its environs.

The Balint groups:

There were 8 and 7 participants in two Balint groups with 2 credentialed leaders per group. The membership of the groups remained the same throughout the trip and we had 100%
participation for all ten sessions over the 5 days. Groups were led in the usual manner, 1 hour groups with consistent leadership. We used the push-back method. What made the setting for our Balint Groups unusual, and perhaps unprecedented, was that we were always outdoors, in rain and shine, thunderstorms and wind, with a roaring river close by. Momentum staff put up tarps overhead on rainy days, but otherwise we were in the elements.

The group members were from a variety of professions: medical providers, psychologists, medical education administration, chiropractic, and nursing. Since a number of the participants were in non-clinical educational or administrative roles, their cases dealt with interpersonal and identity issues that arose in their workplaces. The Balint group members engaged quickly and bonded well. Use was made of the obvious metaphors of river, wildlife etc. When the wind and rain started we just pulled the chairs in closer and finished our work. Safety issues and confidentiality felt secure.

Three of the Balint group members brought non-Balint partners who had a wonderful time
working with the river guides, hiking, fishing, etc. while the Balint groups were in session.

There was a large age range in the overall group. As we had hoped, a number of participants
were early in their careers, and the combination of Balint with a wilderness trip was appealing.
We had 4 intrepid folk in their seventies; our youngest members were in their thirties.
Everyone was together 24/7, paddling on the rafts, changing in and out of wetsuits, living in small tents, brushing teeth along the river and using the portable privy set up by the guides at every stop. Leaders and group members were equal participants in the rafting experience and, though the leaders met every day to debrief, there was no social separation between faculty and participants.

On day 3 we had a meeting with all participants and faculty to get feedback on how everyone was doing. For the most part people were happy. Three participants
asked for more free time, with only one daily Balint session. We held the line at two groups a day, but we asked the Momentum expedition leader to try to get us into camp earlier in the afternoons so that people would have more time to relax or do other activities. The participants overall appreciated the meeting and being heard.

There were four significant challenges for participants and leaders alike, many of whom were inexperienced in at least one of the following:
1. The river - there was a new set of skills to be learned regarding dressing for the river, staying
warm, staying in the raft, paddling, climbing in and out of boats and negotiating one steep, rocky bank.
2. Camping - sleeping in a small tent, sometimes with a stranger, negotiating "bio-breaks," keeping gear organized and dry and the extra challenge of having to break camp and set it up again every day. We were on the move!
3. Wilderness - no internet or cell connectivity for 5 days. Distractions created by the elements, the river in the background, wildlife and birds.
4. Balint work for those with no prior Balint experience - about 1/3 of the participants.

The group members handled logistics each in their own way, but everyone adapted to the
challenges and even found them exhilarating, as shown in their evaluations. We had a sense
that depending on each other while on the river, and sharing all aspects of the camp life, added
to bonding in the groups. Likewise, having the groups as a grounding place made life on the

river that much more enjoyable.

We did have one issue in one of the Balint groups. Unknown to us during Balint group assignments, a group of friends and co-workers ended up in one Balint group. This made it a little more difficult to gain cohesion for the group as a whole.

Balint Outcomes:
Every participant was able to present at least one case. Strong alliances developed among participants with no one being left out. Working together on the river strengthened the
bonds in the group. Our participant evaluations were glowing and reflect this understanding:

*Words cannot capture the splendor of this experience! It was nothing short of spiritual and incredibly healing for me.*
*Being out in the wilderness, free of distractions and doing unfamiliar things with people I didn't know was incredibly freeing and helped us establish even stronger connections than we normally would.*
*I have only ever had wonderful experiences in Balint events. This was the most wonderful!*
*Felt more intense and meaningful sharing time both in Balint and on the river.*
*It was incredible having wilderness as part of the Balint experience; perfect combination.*
*The camaraderie was comparable to intensives and was heightened by the beauty of nature and the time we spent together on the river.*
*The river and our days of adventure did provide us with a plethora of metaphors!*
*This was an exceptional experience. The wilderness setting added unique challenges and opportunities to the Balint process.*

Lessons learned:

1. It is critical to have at least one Balint faculty who is very familiar with the setting.
2. It is important that pre-event information as far as logistics, gear, and what to expect be as complete as possible. This is so important; we all know what to bring for a conference in a hotel, but it's a different matter preparing for the wilderness.
3. We found it important at the beginning of the trip to ensure that participants felt comfortable with setting up and adjusting their gear; this includes tents, wet suits, and safety gear on boats.
4. A congenial, close working relationship between the expedition leaders and the Balint Leaders was very important.
5. The unique setting for the work did obviate the importance of maintaining the usual Balint boundaries including keeping group membership constant, holding to the number of sessions detailed in the event announcement and stressing between- group confidentiality.
6. Daily debriefs for leaders are important to keep track of the groups and foster mutual support among the leaders.

7. We found it important to keep open communications with the expedition leadership daily regarding river-related logistics and plans.

## Conclusions

We believe this trip was incredibly successful. The river experience was thrilling for all the participants, as judged by the evaluations. The Balint experience in this unique setting was true to Balint traditions and was meaningful to people new to the work as well as to experienced Balinters. The wilderness river experience and Balint work were mutually enriching.

The feedback from participants of this event was overwhelmingly positive. Although the event was conceived as a way to hold Balint groups in a wilderness setting, questions arise regarding whether the favorable resultant responses were specific to the wilderness and whether the necessity of learning new, unrelated skills juxtaposed to the Balint sessions might have been part of what made the experience so compelling. Would an outdoor setting without the need to learn and apply new skills unrelated to Balint be as successful? Would an indoor setting requiring the mastery of new skills be comparable?

While this could be studied more objectively, it is our opinion that it wasn't so much the learning of new skills by itself that resulted in the enthusiastically positive experience, but rather it was the real challenge of actual physical risk (however mitigated) and the stretching of one's limits and comfort level that left participants with a sense of having mastered both themselves and the demands of the situation, thus enhancing their feelings of accomplishment and camaraderie with fellow registrants. Overcoming adversity, surviving, and thriving are heady feelings.

In addition, several days and nights in the wilderness required 24/7 involvement and presence. There was no "way out" except to see the trip through. The psychological and emotional impact of this may have been in part subconscious, but it surely affected the perception and workings of Balint participation during the trip.

It is also likely that another wilderness setting, more sedate and with less perceived risk to personal physical safety, would not be quite so exhilarating, however any wilderness location can have an invigorating, intoxicating and even spiritual effect on a person that would be hard to replicate indoors or in a public park or other usual human habitat. It is our hope other Balint organizations will take the idea of doing Balint in the Wilderness and create similar opportunities in other parts of the country and the world. Please then invite us along!

# Workshops

# Workshop 1.
# Introducing Balint to Large Groups

## Ritch Addison, PhD
Clinical Professor, UCSF Family and Community Medicine
Professor Emeritus, Sutter Santa Rosa
Family Medicine Residency
Santa Rosa, California, USA
raddison@sonic.net

## Jeffrey L. Sternlieb, PhD
Associate Professor, Lehigh Valley Health Network,
Family Medicine Residency (retired)
Allentown, Pennsylvania, USA
jsternlieb@comcast.net

**Objective:**
Participants will learn a new, additional way of introducing Balint work to large groups, departments, faculties, health centers and other organizations.

Generating interest in and enthusiasm for Balint work is a crucial issue for the sustainability of Balint over time. If Balint work is to continue to grow and develop it is necessary to find creative and effective ways of engaging individuals with no Balint experience.

Balint work is primarily designed as a small group process to explore the complexities of the clinician-patient relationship. Sometimes opportunities arise to introduce Balint to departments, faculties or other large groups. Usually, such demonstrations have been done either by fish bowl, involving an inner participating group and an outer observing group, or by providing a didactic PowerPoint introduction to Balint, or both. Both have experiential limitations for the reaching the desired audience.

However, there is an additional possibility, especially when large groups are involved. This method has been used for up to 80 participants in a variety of settings and with a variety of specialties and organizations. It is a Balint-like large group process that involves every person imagining a clinician-patient relationship, briefly discussing that relationship with one other person, listening to that person's situation, then Balinting a volunteered case in the large group, where the possibility for everyone to participate exists. The leader(s), well versed in structure and crowd control, demonstrating empathy, understanding, compassion, and welcome, facilitate(s) the entire process.

In this interactive, participatory workshop, attendees will be introduced to a method of providing large groups of individuals stimulating and engaging Balint-like experiences. Attendees will participate in each part of the workshop.

Schedule of 90-minute workshop:
Background Frame in Large Group: 10 minutes
Introductory Slides: 5 minutes
Pair and Share Individual Situations: 10 minutes
Volunteer Case Presentation: 8 minutes
Clarifying Questions: 3 minutes
Collaborative Work in the Large Group: 25 minutes
Presenter rejoins and the large group process closes: 5 minutes
Stretch in place and/or Contingency: 4 minutes
Reflection on Process: Comments, Discussion, Application Possibilities: 20 minutes

Finding additional engaging and experiential ways to introduce Balint to large groups of people who have little or no experience with Balint is crucial for generating increased interest and participation in Balint work.

# Workshop 2.
# Discussion Group on Diversity, Equity, and Inclusion in Balint Groups

Lisa Whitten, PhD
Independent Psychologist
Co-Chair ABS Diversity Committee
New York, New York, USA
lisawhittenphd@gmail.com

Phil Phelps, LCSW
President, American Balint Society
Pittsburgh, Pennsylvania, USA
philphelps@icloud.com

This workshop focuses on work in progress. The intention of this workshop is to bring understanding and compassion to the challenges experienced by Balint group leaders and their group members as they identify and work through themes, emotions, and issues related to Diversity, Equity, Inclusion (DEI). Today this is especially difficult because of our current socially polarized environment and "cancel culture."

**Description of the Workshop**
In 2022, the ABS Diversity Committee created an opportunity for the ABS members to discuss the difficulties Balint Leaders and their groups face when trying to identify and process themes related to DEI. In this workshop, a brief history of the ABS Diversity Committee will be presented, as well as how the committee came to create this virtual space to discuss this exceedingly difficult topic. Participants will be invited to discuss, as in the ABS Diversity Committee virtual groups, the complicated dynamics that arise in Balint groups when the Balint case raises issues related to the full range of individual differences and experiences of exclusion and/or inequity. A question the ABS Diversity Committee was trying to address was: how can we help Balint Leaders be better prepared to identify DEI themes, consult to them if appropriate, keep the group safe, and keep the group focused on the Balint group tasks? Participants will be invited to provide their experience as leaders or members of a group in which the case presentation hinted at a DEI theme, whether it was identified or not, and what happened in their experience. The

participants will then be invited to focus on one Balint group experience, ask questions about it, and give answers to the questions related to what may have helped or held back the group from talking about or addressing the issues related to DEI that the case presentation may have implied. The workshop will end with a summary of ideas provided by the participants regarding what may facilitate or hinder a Balint group leader's ability to recognize these themes, consult to them if contextually appropriate, and successfully facilitate the Balint group when the themes are raised. After the summary, the participants will be invited to provide constructive feedback about how to improve leading a discussion group like this one, and how relevant or necessary a group like this may be in their respective communities.

## Learning Objectives

1. Participants will learn a brief history and progress of the ABS Diversity Committee and their project of having regular Virtual Discussion Groups on DEI in Balint Groups.
2. Participants will be invited to discuss, as in the virtual groups, the complicated dynamics that arise in Balint groups when the Balint case raises issues related to the full range of individual differences and experiences of exclusion and/or inequity.
   a. Questions for discussion could be:
      i. How to help the group explore the patient-clinician relationship when issues of diversity and difference arise
      ii. How to help groups dig deeper as safely as possible
      iii. How to facilitate a group in which the case exposes a risk of exclusion for one of the members or the presenter
      iv. When do you break the Balint frame to keep the group safe and talk about what happened in the group?
3. Participants will provide their assessment and areas of improvement for the Discussion Groups.

## Time Schedule

0:00   Introduction of speakers and quick survey of group, depending on the size.
0:10   Goals and structure of the workshop
            Brief history of the Diversity Committee
            Share Diversity Committee mission statement
            Brief history and development of the discussion group
0:25   Group Discussion
1:15   Feedback and Conclusions
1:25   Give link to brief feedback survey.

# Workshop 3.
# From the Head to the Heart: Cultivating Self-Compassion to Transform Difficult Balint Moments

Renske van den Brink
Medical Doctor and Counsellor
MBchB, DipObs (University of Auckland), FRNZCGP, DipCounseling, NZAC, PGDipHSc(Mind Body Healthcare)
New Zealand
renske42@gmail.com

As a Balint leader, on a good day I can make use of my knowledge and experience even when there is a difficult moment in the group that pushes my buttons. I can notice it is happening, name it silently to myself and choose a wise response to align with the needs of the group. However, if I am tired, stressed or perhaps upset about some other unresolved matter, I am more likely to default to an unconscious reaction such as degrees of internal judgement towards myself or others, an unnecessarily overprotective response (perhaps to relieve my own anxiety), or unconsciously colluding with a group enactment.

This pattern is common and in fact hardwired into us as human beings, due to our evolutionary need to prioritise survival. If there is a threat, all thoughts of care and concern for those around us go out the window. Our first priority is to either oppose the threat by fighting (maybe engaging in verbal debate), fleeing (perhaps withdrawing with silence), or at worst, we might freeze in a dissociative shock reaction.

Self-compassion is an internal self-soothing technique that can powerfully mitigate these tendencies, by creating a more supportive, encouraging and reassuring internal environment during times of internal psychological challenge. Thus, we can rapidly shift the sense of perceived danger back to safety. Self-compassion can be learned even by those of us who have high levels of self-criticism and perfectionism, and evidence abounds to support it's effectiveness particularly in the relevant areas of post-traumatic stress, anxiety and improving the practical aspects of leadership (Neff, K, 2023; Klodiana, L etal, 2021).

In this workshop I will begin with a short 15-minute PowerPoint presentation to cover the basics of self-compassion evidence-based theory. During the remaining 75 minutes, there will be time for supported self-reflection and participants will evaluate their own baseline capacity and tendencies using the self-compassion scale (Neff, K 2022). They will have the opportunity to engage in a practical Balint informed self-reflection exercise to create a context for using self-compassion, and then learn the technique using two stacked self compassion practices. There will be generous opportunity for sharing and discussion to support the practical application of the technique in our Balint work, including an opportunity to explore personal roadblocks which might make self-compassion difficult to learn.

| Time | Task topic | Content | Process |
|------|-----------|---------|---------|
| 15 mins | Teaching theory | Introduction, context, relevant evidence-based research and methods. | Short powerpoint with a resources list. |
| 15 mins | Setting the scene in a Balint group | Reflect and discuss examples of difficult Balint moments (personal or observed) | Think-Pair-Share. Reflection and discussion. |
| 10 mins | What is my current capacity for self-compassion? | An opportunity to evaluate own capacity for self-compassion currently. | Fill in and score the Self-Compassion Scale questionnaire. |
| 20 mins | Practice the foundation skills | Learn and practice the skills of:<br>- somatic awareness<br>- connecting with common humanity<br>- experiencing a felt sense of comfort. | Self-compassion practice 1 (self-reflective and discussion) |
| 20 mins | Practice the applied skills | Apply the above steps to a personal difficult moment | Self-compassion practice 2 (private) |
| 10 mins | Common roadblocks and challenges | Question and answer opportunity to discuss application to our Balint work. | Group discussion |

## References

Klodiana, L. (2021). When Leader Self-Care begets Other Care: Leader Role Self-Compassion and helping at Work. Journal of Applied Psychology, Online First Publication, October 14, 2021. http://dx.doi.org/10.1037/apl0000957.

Neff, K. D. (2023). Self-Compassion: Theory, Method, Research, and Intervention. Annual

Review of Psychology, 74:193-217.

Neff, K. D. & Tóth-Király, I (2022). Self-Compassion Scale (SCS), In N. Oleg, O. N. Medvedev,
C. U. Krägeloh, R. J. Siegert, & N. N. Singh (Eds.) Handbook of Assessment in Mindfulness. New York: Springer. DOI: 10.1007/978-3-030-77644-2_36-1

# Workshop 4.
# Balint and Visual Thinking Strategies

## James Deming, MD
Department of Hospice and Palliative Care
Mayo Clinic Health System – Northwest Wisconsin (retired)
Eau Claire, Wisconsin, USA
deming.james@icloud.com

## Allison K. Bickett, PhD, MS
Department of Family Medicine
Assistant Professor, Wake Forest University School of Medicine
Charlotte, North Carolina, USA
allison.bickett@atriumhealth.org

## Alan Ng Cheng Hin, MBChB, MRCGP, CCFP, FCFP, MMEd
Department of Family Medicine
Assistant Professor, University of Ottawa
Ottawa, Ontario, Canada
ang@uottawa.ca

For decades, art has been incorporated into medical education as a way to foster creative thinking and for developing the human side of training (1). In keeping with the conference goal of using Balint to cultivate compassion and understanding, we propose a 90-minute workshop on Visual Thinking Strategies (2), a well-established structure for promoting understanding of visual art, and the Balint method.

Some Balint leaders have employed Visual Thinking Strategies just before their group session to "prime the pump," give permission to wonder, and encourage divergent thinking (as opposed to the convergent thinking that dominates medical training) (3). This workshop would allow participants to experience the effectiveness of VTS and relate it to their Balint work.

A small portion of the workshop (about 15 minutes) would be didactic, explaining the history and method of Visual Thinking Strategies, which was developed to maximize museum visits and has been shown to stimulate the imagination, promote group learning, and prod articulate expression of different viewpoints.

The framework of VTS is simple, consisting of three questions: 1) What's going on in this picture? 2) What do you see that makes you say that? And 3) What more can we find? There are no wrong answers. Everyone's views are accepted. Group members learn from each other.

Most of the time in the workshop would be spent viewing, as a group, a small selection of visual art, about 15 minutes per piece. The group would be encouraged to discuss the artwork using the VTS framework, and then, with each piece, the group would be asked to reflect on how this VTS experience might influence a Balint group if one were held immediately afterwards.

While Visual Thinking Strategies has enthusiastic supporters, there are others who point out its limits and negative ramifications when used with Balint groups. All viewpoints will be welcomed in our workshop discussion.

Some attendees may emerge as enthusiasts of Visual Thinking Strategies in Balint while others may rule it out. Either way, this session will allow participants to experience the beauty of visual arts and the fun of cooperative learning while deepening their understanding of different ways that Balint may cultivate compassion and understanding.

Objectives: At the end of this workshop, participants should be able to:
1. Define Visual Thinking Strategies and be able to apply it to visual art.
2. Name benefits of weaving education about visual arts into medical education.
3. Relate the potential benefits and drawbacks to incorporating VTS into traditional Balint group sessions.

**References**
1. Dalia Y, Milam EC, Rieder EA. Art in Medical Education: A Review. J Grad Med Educ. 2020 Dec;12(6):686-695. doi: 10.4300/JGME-D-20-00093.1. Epub 2020 Dec 2. PMID: 33391592; PMCID: PMC7771590.
2. Yenawine P. Visual Thinking Strategies: Using Art to Deepen Learning Across School Disciplines. 2018 Harvard Education Press.
3. Hall, M. (2020). Balint autobiography—Mary Hall. The International Journal of Psychiatry in Medicine, 55(3), 207-209. https://doi.org/10.1177/0091217420919016

# Workshop 5.
# Balint Groups in Times of Turmoil:
# To Have or Not to Have?
# Covid-19, War Times, Natural Disasters,
# and other Collective Trauma Situations

## Aya Biderman, MD
Family Physician, Clalit Health Care – Sothern District
Faculty of Health Sciences, Ben-Gurion University of the Negev
Beer Sheva, Israel
abid@bgu.ac.il

## Yuval Shorer, MD
Department of Psychiatry, Soroka Medical Center
Faculty of Health Sciences, Ben-Gurion University of the Negev
Beer Sheeva, Israel
yuvalshorer@gmail.com

## Ruth Kannai, MD
Family Physician, Clalit Health Care – Jerusalem District
Faculty of Health Sciences, Ben-Gurion University of the Negev
Beer Sheeva, Israel
rkannai@gmail.com

## Mark Budow, MD
Family Physician, Clalit Health Care –Dan-Petach-Tikva District
Faculty of Medicine, Tel Aviv University
Tel Aviv, Israel
markb1@bezeqint.net

We invite delegates from all countries who are ready to share their experiences as Balint Group leaders and participants in times of crisis.

## NO MAN IS AN ISLAND John Donne

No man is an island,
Entire of itself,
Every man is a piece of the continent,
A part of the main.
If a clod be washed away by the sea,
Europe is the less.
As well as if a promontory were.
As well as if a manor of thy friend's
Or of thine own were:
Any man's death diminishes me,
Because I am involved in mankind,
And therefore never send to know for whom the bell tolls;
It tolls for thee.

## Introduction (15 minutes)

During the Covid-19 epidemic, the whole world and the health care system experienced a state of turmoil, with anxiety, panic, and uncertainty. Not only the new disease, but also the restrictions put upon people, were a source of suffering and distress. During those days, BALINT GROUPS (BGs) were held in different forms. We had more and more zoomed BGs, and specific issues have risen.

Here are some citations from BGs during the Covid-19 period:

> The leader of a group for residents: "There's a group member missing in the Zoom square today, do I need to call him now to ask if he is OK? Is this my task as a leader?"
> A family physician member: "Since the beginning of the epidemic, I stopped seeing patients in my clinic. You know, my husband's immune system is problematic, and I am afraid to bring the Corona into our home."
> A leader of family medicine residents: "If we don't have a real face-to-face BG, I am not willing to have it through zoom. I won't agree to do BGs by zoom!"

Other examples of collective turmoil include natural disasters, inner political conflicts, and war. In the 7/10/23 war in Israel, BG leaders had a zoom meeting, about 2 months after the war began.

> "…W.T.F  Balint now?!.... Can we have BGs during this time? I am barely balancing my life these days. Have no brain to have BGs!"

"The Balint method is like an old concept. We need to renew it. It doesn't fit our group needs now. I mourn the Balint tool...."

"I'm torn between my "functioning" side of me and the shocked, overwhelmed side of me."

"I'm trying to form a new BG, but the young doctors asked me: Do you want us to present a case of common cold now?!"

"I feel that words will not change a thing today ... "

From these citations, we began to uncover the dilemmas around BGs in times of turmoil. In this workshop, we will think about and share our experiences and stories, in a calm atmosphere.

**Workshop outline**:

For the sake of intimacy and openness, we will start working in small groups (4-6 participants), around these issues:

1. Have you had a dilemma whether to attend or to hold a BG or not? When, why, what happened?

2. As a leader, how would you react if a participant brings up his/her own feelings related to the collective crisis situation and not a case of doctor-patient relations?

3. How did the crisis affect the setting of Balint meetings?

(45 minutes)

Back in the large group, we will ask all groups to summarize and present their thoughts and ideas. Then we will discuss the changes in your Balint Group during the turmoil situation, both as a leader and as a participant.

You can use words or sentences from "NO MAN IS AN ISLAND" or any other poem/song, to bring ideas for dealing with Balint Groups in times of crisis. (30 minutes)

**Learning objectives**: In this workshop participants will

- Share their own experiences as leaders and members of BGs in times of turmoil.
- Discuss the possible modifications needed in BGs during these situations.
- Examine what the phrase "no man is an island" means for them.
- Appreciate the closeness and the similarities of their respective experiences.

# Workshop 6.
# Creating an International Study Design for Measuring the Effects of Balint Groups

Eddo de Lang, MD
Retired Family Physician
Mary Washington Family Medicine Residency Program
Fredericksburg, VA, USA
Wright Center for Graduate Medical Education
National Family Medicine Residency
Washington, DC, USA
eddo.delang@gmail.com

James Deming, MD
Retired Family Physician
Department of Hospice and Palliative Care
Mayo Clinic Health System – Northwest Wisconsin
Eau Claire, Wisconsin, USA
deming.james@icloud.com

This is a proposal to conduct an international study to measure the long-term effects of attending Balint Groups by comparing different parameters in populations that do and do not participate in Balint Groups. Those who have been active in Balint have experienced that the Balint method can be a powerful tool to cultivate understanding and compassion. This comparative study seeks to document the effects of Balint groups and hopefully create a strong case for others to support them.

## Background

In the past years, there have been several attempts to show the positive effects of Balint Group participation. The Scholarly Activity Committee of the American Balint Society is designing a descriptive study to demonstrate an increase in empathy in those who participate in Balint Groups in the US.

To take this one step further we would like to design a multi-year comparative international study that hopefully will be able to show several benefits of participation in Balint Groups, compared with non-Balint participants. The study could for example look at changes in levels of empathy, burn-out, job satisfaction and self-perception. Depending on the study design we may be able to show differences in change for different corners of the globe.

During this workshop we would like to create an environment wherein we can construct a study design together. We very much would like to poll the opinions of different professions from different backgrounds to create a meaningful study design that would answer most questions each one of us could have. We realize that the questions we have may vary depending on the discipline, cultural background, and levels of curiosity of the attendants in this workshop and that is exactly what we are looking for: diversity of thoughts and expectations, just like a Balint Group.

## Design of the workshop:

1. Introduction: a brief (10 to 15-minute) discussion explaining the concepts of the proposed study.
2. Subgroups: after the introduction each subgroup will tackle different questions (20-30 minutes).
3. The outcome: each subgroup's conclusions will be brought to the large group for a final discussion with the goal of summarizing the findings and creating a wishlist of all the elements we created together to be used as the framework for the study design. (45 minutes)

4. Invitation:

Those who are interested in this study concept and who have the time to further developing it and perhaps later even with the execution of the plans are welcome to join us to turn this speculation into reality.

# Workshop 7.
# The Shape of Empathy,
# an Exploration of Body and Imagination

## Kris Wheeler, MA
Private Practice
Faculty, Center for Object Relations
Seattle, Washington, USA
kris@kriswheeler.com

A Balint Group asks participants to consider what it may feel like to be the presented patient and what it might feel like to be the provider. Elaboration generally moves in the direction of reflecting on emotional life. This workshop will support participants to open their imaginations into the experiences of others through somatic embodiment.

Neuroscience research indicates the existence of circuits in the brain that mediate somatic embodiment of other people in our own bodies. These circuits appear to allow us to directly experience the behavioral impulses and emotional states of other people. Such merger phenomena give information to the intuitive and creative capacities we possess in the context of a patient/provider interaction.

I was a professional dancer and dance educator and once a dancer, always a dancer! Over the subsequent decades, I have integrated my love of movement into my healing work. The conference theme of compassion and understanding inspires me to submit this workshop for your consideration.

This workshop offers the opportunity to be literal about the metaphor of standing in the shoes of another. I will facilitate an awareness and movement process designed to support participants to experience what it feels like to be another by placing their whole body in the posture and gestures of another.

The design of the workshop will begin with a mindfulness-like process of helping participants attune to their somatic experience. I will guide a practice that directs attention to shifts in body alignment/posture and to the organic movement of arms and hands. This somatic awareness gives rise to images and memories about these inner experiences of postural and gestural shifts. Images and memories in turn prompt further shifts in movement, and a movement exploration ensues that has a reflective quality of understanding and compassion.

Participants may take this opportunity to feel what it is like to live in the body of one person they care about, perhaps a patient or family member. This involves the ability to experience the rhythms of that person's breathing, the patterns of tensions in that person's face, the energetic impulses in their body, the dynamic forces that flow through their body as they adapt to gravity while they move in the world. Alternatively, rather than focus on a single person, participants may simply find ways to loosen their grip on their own somatic signature and find a fluidity that supports a greater capacity to experience of states of being than is typical of them.

I will utilize the format of Authentic Movement, a widely known and practiced somatic embodiment method, in which movers work with their eyes closed to the extent they are comfortable. This method generally supports the experience of being deeply internal as well as subtle.

After about 45 minutes of attention to movement we will pair up for discussion to harvest what was gleaned. The final 10-15 minutes will be a full group circle to collect the group's reflection on this experience.

Learning goals:

1. Participants will gain greater awareness of their own posture and their characteristic movement signature.
2. Participants will increase their understanding of how posture and movement of the body, especially the spine, influences the experience of identity and suggests options for elaboration of one's identity.
3. Participants will increase ways to identify with and understand another's experience of living in the particular configuration of a body other than one's own.

# Workshop 8.
# Research cum Training – ABS Style

## Jeffrey L. Sternlieb, PhD
Associate Professor, Lehigh Valley Health Network,
Family Medicine Residency (retired)
Allentown, Pennsylvania, USA
jsternlieb@comcast.net

## Ritch Addison, PhD
Clinical Professor, UCSF Family and Community Medicine
Professor Emeritus, Sutter Santa Rosa Family Medicine
Residency
Santa Rosa, California, USA
raddison@sonic.net

**Objective:**

Participants will experience a deeper exploration of some of the dynamics in doctor-patient relationships through their participation in written reflection followed by their group's discussion of this process, its impact and its potential.

The most frequently prescribed medicant is the doctor him or herself, according to Michael Balint (1957, p. 4). However, little was known (in 1957) about the pharmacology of this drug. This is the subject of the rest of <u>The Doctor, His Patient and the Illness</u>, along with the four subsequent books that report on multi-year study groups conducted in the now familiar 'research cum training' process that is Balint.

Many medical professionals who are new to participating in Balint groups appreciate the experience in their Balint group; however, they are often baffled at the end of the group. With no conclusion or answer or some sort of ending, there are no suggestions for using or somehow benefiting from that experience. More experienced professionals are less uncomfortable with endings based on time and not solutions. However, what do we do with or how do we process the various contributions to the group's understanding of the case that was presented?

Much of what we understand about doctor-patient relationships comes from study groups begun and modeled by Michael Balint. The members of these groups were also the researchers. The research consisted of Michael and Enid Balint's distillation of the multiple discussions about the cases that were presented as well as follow up reports about previously presented cases. In other words, Balint's participants in his study groups reflected on and wrote about their reflections about their cases.

Most Balint group participants have many thoughts and emotions stirred up during the discussion of a case, their own or others' cases. However, there have been few systematic opportunities to reflect on the group process or to write about those reflections or to discuss either their thoughts or any new awareness. Without this processing, we leave too much material about our own pharmacology "on the proverbial table!"

In this workshop, the goal is to demonstrate a method of developing a deeper understanding of the doctor-patient dynamics as revealed by a Balint group that is followed by a structured writing and discussion debrief.:

- We will introduce and explain the process:
    - participants will participate in a typical Balint group.
    - At the completion of the case discussion, participants will be invited to begin writing their own thoughts or personal reflections about the Balint group discussion in which they participated.
- Any and all written reflections may be kept private.
- A discussion focused on this reflective process will follow.
- The two groups together will continue the discussion, including creating opportunities for future processing of Balint group experiences.
- We will end with a reminder of Balint's original goal of developing one's own pharmacology as a frequently prescribed drug.

11:00 - 11:10 Brief Introduction

11:10 - 11:55 Balint group

11:55 - 12:05 writing reflections

12:05 - 12:20 group and writing debrief

12:20 - 12:30 future opportunities for "mining" the Balint group experience

# Posters

# Establishing Balint Group for Third Year Medical Students and Evaluating Its Impact on Burnout, Empathy, Resilience and Strength of Motivation – A Preliminary Qualitative Analysis

Authors: Dr Ignazio Graffeo, Dr Angela Kearns, Dr Sabina Fahy, Dr Peter Humphries, Dr Ronan Byrne, Dr Ramona Novac, Dr Ahmad Iqbal, Dr Patricia Marley, Dr Patricia Noonan, Helen Clark, Prof Dimitrios Adamis, Prof Geraldine McCarthy
Corresponding Author: Dr Ignazio Graffeo, Sligo/Leitrim Mental Health Services – graffeoignazio@yahoo.it and Ignazio.graffeo@hse.ie
Affiliations: Sligo/Leitrim Mental Health Services, Donegal Mental Health Services, Mayo Mental Health Services, Galway Mental Health Services, Galway School of Medicine, Sligo University Hospital Library

## ABSTRACT

Healthcare professionals in Ireland today are required to work in highly challenging settings.
Preparing medical students to develop resilience and acquire the skills to cope with these circumstances is difficult, even before the pandemic. Reflective practice for medical students aims to provide them with the means to process and manage some of the challenges they will face in the workplace. The principal aims of this research are to improve medical students' well-being and support system, to ascertain the difference in scoring of four questionnaires, to understand if there is an objective and quantifiable increase in empathy, resilience and motivation and a decrease in burnout levels and to analyse the feedback provided by the students. This is a cohort prospective study across four academic sites aimed at assessing the response of third-year medical students in four areas of interest (burnout, empathy, resilience, strength of motivation), before and after receiving a six-week course of Balint group. Students were also asked to complete an evaluation form at the end of the reflective practice course. The research type is mixed quantitative and qualitative.

# What Do Some Balint Leadership Intensive Participants Say During Their Experience?

Author: Barbara Hemmendinger, MSS, CBL
Affiliations: Associate Director/Behavioral Science, Williamsport Family Medicine Residency, Williamsport, Pennsylvania, USA (retired).
bhemmend@aol.com.

**ABSTRACT**

Acquiring knowledge and skills are significant aspects of the American Balint Society's Intensive Leadership training, and being immersed in six Balint group sessions over a four-day period develops experiential and emotional learning. Having generated a word cloud for this poster presentation, we will display commonalities derived from the de-identified reactions to the training shared by nine participants who formed a convenience sample and were individually videorecorded during the penultimate day of a recent in-person leadership Intensive. Using content analysis, we will also examine differences and similarities between those participants who had never previously attended an Intensive and those who already had prior Intensive experience.

The poster will also contain a QR code that links to a short ABS video featuring clips excerpted from the participants described above.

# Balint Groups and Health Professionals' Perceived Well-Being – An Israeli Study

Authors: Ruth Kannai MD, Aya Biderman MD, Tamar Freud PhD, Shai Krontal MD

Corresponding author: Ruth Kannai MD rkannai@gmail.com

Affiliations: Health Services and Ben-Gurion University of the Negev, Faculty of Health Sciences, Department of Family Medicine; Siall Research Center for Family Medicine and Primary Care; Haim Doron Division of Community Health

Beer Sheva, Israel; Department of Family Medicine, Maccabi Healthcare Services

Department of Family Medicine, Faculty of Medicine, Tel Aviv University, Tel Aviv, Israel

## ABSTRACT

Health professionals' well-being is a goal that impacts patients' care, their satisfaction and outcomes. Previous studies that have demonstrated the positive effects of Balint Groups (BGs) are descriptive and based on small sample sizes. We evaluated the perceptions of health professionals who participated in BGs, to identify the factors related to their perceived well-being.

In January and February 2023, we performed a cross-sectional study. We distributed a questionnaire to members of the Israeli internet network of Family physicians, to a mailing list of the Israeli BG association and during a conference for Family Medicine teachers. The questionnaire included demographic and professional information and a 5-point Likert scale for the level of agreement with a list of 15 statements regarding BGs. We received 142 responses, most of whom were family physicians. More than half were teachers and/or leaders in the medical system.

Respondents who had participated in BGs reported a reduction in burnout, increased empathy, enhanced professional identity and better relationships with patients and colleagues. Those who attended BGs for more than 5 years reported significantly more positive outcomes compared to those who attended less than 1 year. In a logistic regression analysis, we found two factors significantly associated with self-reported well-being: attending BGs for more than five years and perceiving BGs as a means for relieving burnout. Participation in BGs seems to have a positive impact on healthcare professionals' perceived well-being and professional development. The findings suggest that medical organizations should encourage the regular availability of BGs to support health professionals' well-being.

# An Approach to the Establishment of Online Balint Groups for Medical Students across the United States

Authors: Leah Kunins, BS; Kaylea Horacek, BS

Corresponding Author: leah.kunins@ufl.edu; khoraceck@une.edu

Affiliations: University of Florida College of Medicine, Gainesville, Florida, USA (LK); University of New England College of Osteopathic Medicine, Biddeford, Maine, USA (KH)

## ABSTRACT

In the United States, there are currently only a handful of medical schools that currently incorporate Balint training into undergraduate medical education. For those medical schools, Balint training is typically done within the institution and is limited to matriculants. This poster outlines an approach to the development of online Balint groups for medical students from a variety of schools across the United States. The process of identifying and recruiting interested medical students through cold emailing Deans of Medical Education at 155 US accredited medical schools is outlined. The organization of 6 online groups of 10-12 medical students, 2 Student Liaisons, and 2 faculty leaders established a framework for the future of Balint within undergraduate medical education.

# Notes

# Notes

# Notes

# Notes

# Notes

Made in United States
Troutdale, OR
09/27/2024

23200256R00097